PRAISE FOR THE GIFT OF MORE

"When the hard realities of this life strike at your own family ... your own son, even wandering souls will reach out to the divine for answers to the unavoidable and unacceptable. *The Gift of More* shares a mother's inspirational journey from anguish and the challenging limitations of modern health care, to a greater faith through a miraculous intervention from above."

—Ron Panzer
President
Hospice Patients Alliance

"Sean Reynolds' death seemed as improbable as it was painful at the end, but it was also a life-sustaining spiritual journey for Pam Yates, the mother who worked tirelessly to give him as much time and as many choices as possible. *The Gift of More* is truly a love story that will give readers the hope they need in their own lives."

—Mark Hare
Metro Columnist
Rochester *Democrat and Chronicle*

"I read *The Gift of More* while undergoing chemotherapy. It touched my heart. *The Gift of More* will remind you that life is truly a gift, and to love, laugh, and have faith everyday—no matter what!"

—Christi LoTempio
Cancer Survivor

"As a world traveler and a seeker of spiritual wisdom, I consider myself fortunate to know Pamela Yates. Her ability to communicate her quest for wholeness, her own and humanity's, reminds us that we have the power to make as well as see rainbows.

How honored the reader of *The Gift of More* is ... to share travel toward insight with Pamela as she communes questions and revelations. She guides us gently to teach us that real religious feeling is, in fact, the spontaneous growth of sensitive living in the here and now."

—Leslie Kennedy
TV and PR consultant

"Pam Yates is extraordinary. In fact, on my radio show I refer to her as 'one of the world's great women.' Her zest for life is apparent. She earns that accolade as a wife, a friend, and most of all, a mother. When you read of her strength and courage in saying the final goodbye to her 25-year-old son Sean, you'll see for yourself just how extraordinary she is."

—Sandy Beach
WBEN
Buffalo, NY

"A mother's gift to the world is her loving children. Pam's gift to loving parents is her personal account of undying love.

I can't think of another book that better illustrates the transition of grief to comfort and peace."

—Linda Pellegrino
Channel 7
Buffalo, NY

THE
GIFT
OF
MORE

THE GIFT OF MORE

Lessons of faith and love from a life cut short.

Pamela Yates

a memoir

FaithWalk
PUBLISHING

Grand Haven, Michigan

Scripture quotations are taken from the Holy Bible, King James Version, Cambridge, 1769.

Printed in the United States of America
10 09 08 07 06   7 6 5 4 3 2

Library of Congress Cataloging-in-Publication Data

Yates, Pamela, 1945-
  The gift of more / Pamela Yates.—1st ed.
      p. cm.
   ISBN-13: 978-1-932902-46-4 (pbk.)
   ISBN-10: 1-932902-46-5
   1. Suffering—Religious aspects—Christianity. 2. Consolation. 3. Mothers—Religious life. 4. Children—Death—Religious aspects—Christianity. 5. Cancer—Religious aspects—Christianity. I. Title.
   BV4909.Y38 2005
   248.8'6—dc22
                              2005013384

To my mother, Rose.
For her strength, wisdom, and great humanity.

TABLE OF CONTENTS

FOREWORD

It is said that nothing can be more traumatic for an adult than the loss of a child. Moreover, it borders on the impossible to believe that such a tragedy can be the source of inspiration and a strange, mysterious contact with higher powers.

I was involved with such a phenomenon in the autumn of 1994 when my beloved stepson, Sean Reynolds, died in our arms after a long and courageous battle against a rare form of cancer. While I played a supporting role in the tragedy, I witnessed the strength and courage of my wife Pamela, who not only stood steadfastly in support of Sean, hour by hour, day by day, during his agonizing and painful decline, but, following his death, garnered the inner strength to write this chronicle—a passionate yet powerful journal of the events that led us, in the wake of our loss, to find inspiration and hope.

Where most people might be expected to crumble in the face of such heartache and loss, Pamela found a mysterious kind of divine inspiration in the midst of her trial. Having experienced the incident that magnifies and enhances this otherwise painful experience, Pamela found the raw bravery to chronicle the following in her own words. A woman of great talent as a former professional singer and successful businesswoman, she had never written anything more involved than a college term paper. Yet she composed the story that follows with admirable skill. As a professional writer, I was prepared to edit and modify her material, but instead discovered that with her innate skills with the English language the words fell easily on the page and needed little or no tuning.

The result is a story of personal power and inspiration that transcends the shattering loss of our son and—through a flash of mystery and an expression of humanity and strength—brings hope and faith to all who read it.

Brock Yates
Wyoming, New York

ACKNOWLEDGMENTS

Having spent so many years in the writing of this book, I am compelled to remember and thank all the people who have traveled on this journey with me. The obvious ones appear on the pages that follow. As I recalled each person, I began to see my life as one large, unfinished mosaic. Each encounter with a person, be it good or bad, placed a piece in the picture. Each piece was vital to the whole. Every encounter lent strength and structure to an unknowable finished work. I came to believe that each person I met along the way contributed to the tools and skills I needed to master the trials that life has put before me.

Therefore, to all the people who have touched my life, positively or negatively, my undying gratitude. Nothing has been easy about this book. Not in the living, not in the writing, and not in the publishing. The publishing has been a strange story in and of itself. So, thanks to Debra Hampton and John Sprague, formerly of Thomas More Publishing, for their support and encouragement. To the ever there Dirk Wierenga of FaithWalk Publishing, for his deep commitment to our story. He has been a true mentor. A special thanks to William Brown, my sensitive and thoughtful editor. I know the manuscript was a hard one to work on, but his calm and gentle way helped me craft this most difficult project. For helping to give birth to my story, Ginny McFadden and Louann Werksma of FaithWalk Publishing. To our agent Jim Fitzgerald, who took a giant leap from representing "guy books" to finding a home for this distinctly different story. Sean and I will be forever in his debt.

For reasons of personal privacy and legal complications, many names of people, and those of some institutions, have been changed. With approval, certain names have remained unchanged because I wanted them to be honored for their significant roles in this story.

To our friends who loved and supported us through our ordeal and who grace our lives still: Scott and Susan Hill, Ross and Paula Sherwood, Adriana Betts, Bill and Lynn Neal, and Wayne and Linda Purdy.

To Barbara Bramer, our secretary at the time of Sean's illness, who handled all the details of our careers so that I could concentrate on Sean. She was truly an angel sent from heaven, a special person at a special time. To Gayle Young and Jessica Baltz, who contributed their time and energies in the typing of the manuscript. To Stephanie Santiago, a second daughter, for her love and care for us. To my good friend and assistant Melissa Allen, who never let me give up and has helped me in ways she can never fully know.

To my mother and father for always being with me in good times and bad.

To the true champions of our story: Dr. Avrum Bluming and Dr. Robert Nadeau; Cary Milda, R.N., and Betty James, R.N. of Hospice, Batavia, New York; attorney Michael Law, and Chris Reynolds, paralegal, of Phillips, Lytle, Hitchcock, Blaine & Huber, for their commitment to making the world a better place.

For his courage in covering our story, I acknowledge Bob Davis, investigative reporter for *USA Today*. He understood the big picture. To Sandy Beach of WBEN talk radio, Buffalo; Linda Pellegrino of AM Buffalo; WKBW TV; Mark Hare, columnist for the Rochester *Democrat and Chronicle*; and Roger DuPuis II, *Batavia Daily News*, Batavia, New York.

Our grandchildren Sarah and Scott, whose love and sweetness fill my life. Our children: Claire, Dan, and Brock, son-in-law Bobby, and daughter-in-law Cyndy, for their love and sense of family. They were there for Sean when he needed them most.

To our precious daughter, Stacy, one of the most courageous and wise people I have ever known.

Last but not least, a loving thanks to my greatest blessing, my husband Brock. Without his belief in me, I could never have put my private thoughts and emotions on paper. It is also because of him that I know the true meaning of unconditional love.

Although the mosaic of my life remains unfinished, I take great comfort in knowing that we shall all meet again.

Pamela Yates
Wyoming, New York
2005

ONE

BEGINNINGS

Life's journey takes us down many roads; some smooth and others, as we say in the country, seasonal and bumpy, and only passable at certain times of the year. Yet all roads lead us somewhere.

One summer morning in late July 1993 was especially sweet, glorious, and lush. The beautiful valley that flowed softly from our front door resembled a giant jewel-toned quilt. The perfectly formed squares of early corn dressed in verdant green were stitched up against golden expanses of wheat, filling the soul with the promise of plenty. The air was still dewy fresh, not yet burning with the midday heat to come. Western New York summer days are the very reason we who live here tolerate all the badmouthing our winters receive from the rest of the country. We are immune to the national news headlines proclaiming that Buffalo and Rochester are being buried in snow. It's all worthwhile to us because, when spring, summer, and fall are here, there is no place on earth more beautiful.

My husband Brock was born and raised in a small city outside of Buffalo. After our marriage, we moved to a new three-story condominium in a trendy, year-round recreation community outside Torrington, Connecticut. Lakeridge, with its environmentally proper architecture was tucked discreetly in the Berkshire Mountains of western Connecticut.

For many families it was a second-home community, and those who purchased there were mostly from New York City. Lakeridge's advertisements in the *New York Times* and *Wall Street Journal* promised the "good life." It was a wakeup call that wasn't wasted on us, especially since we had two young children to keep occupied in a safe environment. It would also ease our guilt at having to leave them so often for business travel. (In those early years we traveled extensively because of Brock's auto racing commentary for CBS sports.) Aside from the beauty of the place, it boasted its own ski slope, a lake, indoor and outdoor swimming pools, equestrian trails, and a couple of fitness centers—perfect solutions for the needs of our newly formed family. We thought our two children, Sean and Stacy, would be so occupied they wouldn't even know we were away. It turned out to be a parental fantasy. After about six months in "paradise," they were bored to death with condo life, and it gave Brock the perfect opportunity to convince us to move to his beloved western New York State.

Brock and I met in the mid 1970s. He was writing for *Car and Driver*, *Sports Illustrated* and *Playboy* magazines. I was freelancing in marketing and publishing. We met at an annual event thrown by *Car and Driver* at Lime Rock, Connecticut. At first it seemed we had nothing in common. Never in a million years would a dating service put us together. Brock is a laid-back Type C personality and I'm a driven Type A. Yet we share some very deep and profound beliefs, and we soon discovered that our approach to life is the same.

So, after our false start in Connecticut, we moved to Wyoming, New York—population 350—halfway between Buffalo and Rochester and in one of the largest agricultural counties in the state. The landscape resembles the countryside of England, with its rolling hills and fertile valleys. We bought a house called Farmstead.

Farmstead was the culmination of the dream of C.B. Matthews, a rival of John D. Rockefeller in the natural gas and petroleum business. Designed in the earlier Federal style, the house reflected the opulence of its era and Matthew's station in the community. Six beautiful fireplaces and breathtaking woodwork adorn its twenty elegant rooms. Once the center of a thousand-acre farm, Farmstead's orchards produced a wide selection of apples that were shipped by the barrel to France. It also boasted the first Black Angus cattle in the area.

In 1909 Matthews hired architect Bryant Fleming, who later founded the School of Landscape Design at Cornell University, to enlarge and remodel the original farmhouse, built in 1822. Fleming and Matthews traveled to Italy in search of light fixtures and other décor for the house. After its renovation in 1910, Farmstead provided shelter and comfort to seven generations of the Matthews family.

With the passing of time, the Matthews family left Farmstead. Yet Farmstead stood straight and proud awaiting its next love affair with a new generation of devoted owners—the Yates family.

As we began *our* process of restoration some seventy years after the Matthews family had put its mark on the house, I realized that my usual impatience and desire to have things done immediately would have to take a backseat to the massive scope of the project. A house that size had its own timetable. I began to think in terms of normal time versus "Farmstead time." Farmstead time was slower, more thoughtful—and demanded our full attention. The exquisitely detailed carved moldings, the positioning of the rooms, the badly damaged silver platings on the lighting fixtures and the elegant glass sconces all needed special craftsmen to refurbish them. The attention to detail employed in creating this special house had to be respected.

The calming, old-world atmosphere that Farmstead exuded was a stark contrast to my childhood years. As the only child of a successful but alcoholic father, I lived with a daily diet of tension and high drama. My mother tried to create a sense of normalcy for my sake, but with little success.

I quickly learned the child-of-alcoholics' coping skills of seesawing between parents. Without other siblings to buffer the pain and confusion, I would yo-yo back and forth, trying to placate and accommodate the two people I loved most. I became the shock absorber for the emotional chaos that engulfed and immobilized our small family unit. Maintaining the equilibrium and stretching out the good times became my most desperate preoccupation. The angst caused by loving both of my parents and not knowing what I could do to make them happy overshadowed all of my childhood days. For a while I believed that if I behaved better and was more successful, I could fix the broken parts of my family.

The strongest bond my father and I shared was our love and appreciation for music. A frustrated band singer, he and my mother worked hard to help me develop my musical talents and aspirations. The one thing that they did share deeply was a belief that I could accomplish anything I put my mind to. Because that seemed to make them as happy as they could be together, I tried always to succeed and bring them some joy. Their loving faith in me was a gift that I'll always cherish.

My teenage years, although lonely, were filled with endless singing, dancing, and acting lessons. Through hard work and dedication I became part of two summer stock companies: The Lake Placid Playhouse in Lake Placid, New York and the Dorset Playhouse in Dorset, Vermont. Even though I was a good student and my hours were filled with music and theatre, I constantly struggled with the need to do more and make my parents proud. It wasn't until much later that I accepted I was incapable of fixing their problems. Only they could do that.

I met my first husband when I was eighteen and attending Denver University. He was a handsome, bright young man and seemed to be the antithesis of my father. When I brought him home to my parents in New York—to my astonishment—my father liked him. My mother, with her customary sharp instincts, was not so impressed. But since I loved him, she went along—putting my happiness over her instincts.

My father quickly helped him to find a good job in advertising and started molding him into "his kind of guy." The advertising business in the 1960s and 1970s provided good money and lavish perks, and my fiancé found his niche quickly.

We had a big wedding and, from a distance, we looked like the golden couple. We found an apartment in New York City, and a little more than a year later, on January 26, 1967, Sean was born. He was seven pounds of pure sweetness. As an only child I had not had much contact with newborn babies and became fascinated with Sean. He was a miracle. My own personal miracle. With blonde hair, blue eyes, and an engaging smile, he was truly a happy baby who loved to cuddle. My father beamed with joy, and my mother finally had someone to fill the void that my father's drinking had created in her life.

Even though my marriage was rocky from the start, my new little pal compensated for everything. I would take Sean in his stroller and walk the streets of New York to do our family shopping and pass the lonely days. He giggled and brought joy to all he met along the way. When Sean was just months old he would sit in front of the TV watching *Sesame Street*. He loved the music, and together we would sing the songs and laugh at the skits.

When I was in my early twenties and Sean was seven months old I landed a job with Sammy Kaye's orchestra. At the time my husband was out of a job and we needed the money. Working with Sammy Kaye also allowed me to achieve my *father's* lifelong ambition to be a professional singer. I rushed home to my parents to tell them the news. My mother was thrilled and my father wept for joy. I had finally arrived.

Getting the job with Sammy Kaye was one thing, keeping it was another. Kaye hired me on Monday and told me to learn all the music and meet him on Saturday. "Where should I meet you, Mr. Kaye, and when do we rehearse?" I asked.

He snapped, "We don't rehearse. You're a professional aren't you? Meet us on second base at Yankee Stadium for the warm-up show at the Old Timer's game."

I couldn't get out of his door fast enough, trying not to cry like a silly fool in front of him.

I traveled with the orchestra for two years until my daughter Stacy was born. Then I quit to raise my children.

My husband never seemed to be able to hold a job. We moved from New York to a suburb of Philadelphia. It was a fresh beginning where we could own a home and a car. Things went well for a time with my husband's career, and I coped with my babies. As a newborn, Stacy was a handful. Not a bad handful, but definitely not compliant like Sean. Stacy challenged me at every turn. She was sweet and foxy and could manipulate the birds out of the trees. My husband couldn't be counted on, so we three became our own family.

Soon their father was out of work again and we moved to Yorktown Heights, a distant suburb of New York City, where he found a job with *Car and Driver* in the advertising department. The action and energy of New York coupled with the long commute gave him more excuses not to come home to his family. Even though I was unhappy, some of my best memories are of those days, particularly the early evenings.

I would put our favorite songs on the record player and Sean, Stacy, and I would form a conga line going from room to room, singing and dancing our hearts out. When I was younger, I spent all my free time watching movies of old musicals. I had been a Fred Astaire and Gene Kelly addict all my life. The fabulous songs and gloriously elaborate scenes carried me away. In every film, *I* was the girl dancing with Gene and Fred. I became part of the glamorous cast in a world devoted to gentle, sweet camaraderie where every ending was a happy one.

Time passed quickly and, before I knew it, Stacy was two years old and an imp. She looked like a little blonde doll with perfect features. Wearing her favorite long robe, she would try to dance in the conga line, tripping over the robe every few steps. She refused to take it off and spare herself the falls. She loved that robe. I can still see her blond ponytail bobbing up and down as she tried to hold on to Sean. As Stacy tried to grab hold of Sean's waist, he would start to giggle and wiggle his fanny to shake her free. They would collapse with laughter, and the tickling would begin.

Each evening at five o'clock this wonderful music routine would begin, and it would last until around seven, with me knowing that my husband might not make it home. I worked hard to keep the children distracted to blur the realities of our family life and their father's absence. Even though my children brought me great joy, the loneliness and feelings of abandonment were bitterly painful. I was beginning to realize it would be less painful if I were not married.

Our divorce was the scariest decision I ever made. For nine years I had tried to make the marriage work, but my husband just couldn't seem to find his way home at night. The children were getting older and starting to understand and ask questions. I knew if I didn't get out, I might never find happiness for myself or my children. The worst thing I could imagine was arriving bitter at my old age, regretting that I never had the courage to take control of my life and change it.

At thirty-one I became a single parent. I found part-time jobs that I could do at home to make ends meet. I began to hone my sales and marketing skills, which ultimately led me to my meeting and falling in love with Brock.

Once Brock and I married and moved to western New York, it was time to work on blending our two families. Brock's three children—Brock Jr., nineteen (who Brock always called Brocker), Daniel, seventeen, and Claire, fifteen—lived with their mother. Sean and Stacy, who were ten and seven years old, lived with us. The blending of families is rocky at best, and ours was no exception. We talked endlessly about our children and how to do the best we could for each of them. In our case the rural setting was a challenge for my children and me. It was a new world and a dramatic change from our roots in the city. I was used to the theater, shopping, and restaurants. As with most New Yorkers, I had a love-hate relationship with the city. Farmstead was wonderful, but it wasn't

New York City, and the move was particularly hard on the kids. We had also become a curiosity because our move coincided with the release of *Cannonball Run*—the film written by my husband.

Stacy handled it best because she had confidence in herself and made friends easily. Sean, on the other hand, struggled to find his way. He was in junior high, was less outgoing and didn't understand the new culture he was in. Soon both Sean and Stacy opted to go away to boarding school where they could have a wider choice of classes. Earlier Sean had become fascinated with tap dancing. On his tenth birthday, to my joy and amazement, he had asked to take lessons. After we moved to Wyoming, however, he decided it was unmanly to tap dance. When he went away to school he became an accomplished photographer. He was an excellent athlete and played lacrosse.

After Sean and Stacy left for boarding school, I had to find a project or business to keep me challenged. One day, while driving Brock to the airport, we noticed that Wyoming's old hook-and-ladder company was up for sale. It was a brick building, built in 1908. Because of its wonderful period look, it reminded me of one of the most fabulous Christmas shops I had ever seen—Kathe Wholfart in Rothenburg, Germany.

In 1986, the old hook-and-ladder company building became the property of Pamela and Brock Yates. It was a thrilling moment. I felt that if I could create more of an "attraction" with ever-changing displays, people might come from all over and then tell their friends to come, too. The Gaslight Christmas and Holiday Shoppe opened August 1, 1987 and was a great success. But with that success came another problem. How would we feed the people who were coming here? In 1988 we purchased another building in the village square and opened the Cannonball Run Pub and Gaslight Village Café. Other adventurous souls jumped on board and opened shops. Now the village is one of western New York's most beloved tourist destinations. The Gaslight Christmas and Holiday Shoppe, Silas Newell's Provisions, and the Gaslight Village Café & Cannonball Run Pub have been featured on television and radio programs nationwide.

Sean and Stacy would often say, "When mom gets bored—look out!"

In 1992 Sean was a handsome young man of twenty-five. Even with all he had going for himself, I worried about him because he suffered from low self-esteem. Always fascinated by comedy writing and video production, he announced that year that he had talked with the people at The Nashville Network and would be moving to Nashville to begin apprenticing with the TNN film crew. He hoped to carve out a career for himself in television. With mere days to digest Sean's announcement, we wished him well and he was off. We were shocked, proud, happy, and slightly sad. But it was the way Sean did things, and we learned to roll with it.

To our surprise, he not only landed the job but excelled at it. After several months, there was an opening for a production coordinator in Los Angeles for a show called *Truckin' USA* to be hosted by country western singer Ed Bruce. There were two obstacles, however. The position called for someone who could write scripts and type. Sean had never tried either. Yet he was determined. He gathered up dozens of TNN cable shows and bought a computer. He locked himself in his small studio apartment in Nashville and watched countless hours of TNN shows while he taught himself to type. By the end of a month, he had produced a TV script. To the amazement of his bosses at the production company, Sean delivered an excellent script and got the job. He was now the official production coordinator for *Truckin' USA*. Sean had found himself. A promising new career lay ahead. Everything seemed to be going well for him.

For several months, however, Sean had been experiencing lower back pain. He had been working out and lifting heavy camera equipment, so when a highly recommended orthopedist issued a diagnosis of a herniated disc it made sense to everyone. When many more months of pain medication and physical therapy did not relieve the symptoms, Sean's orthopedic surgeon decided that surgery to fix the disc was in order. We spoke with the doctor and his assistant several times and arranged to go to Los Angeles to be with Sean for the surgery and to help with the recovery process. His doctor had the best of credentials, and the surgery went well.

While the prognosis looked good, when I first arrived in L.A. and saw Sean I was stunned at how much weight he had lost. I reasoned that the stress of his new job coupled with the chronic pain must have wreaked havoc on Sean's appetite. I decided to spend several weeks with him as he recuperated and remained until we got the green light from the doctor that Sean could return to work. Finally, the road ahead looked smooth in every direction. At the end of May 1993 I returned to New York, my home and my husband.

On that Saturday morning in July 1993 the warmth and heat of the early morning sun could already be felt through Farmstead's bedroom window. Stacy had just graduated with a bachelor's degree from Ohio Wesleyan University. Sean was finding himself. He was happy with his newfound friends, co-workers, and career. My parents had decided to make a surprise visit from White Plains to spend a week in the country. Brock's wonderful mother was living on her own and still going strong at eighty-six—in the same house after sixty years. His children—Claire, Brocker, and Dan—were living on the west coast and beginning their careers, all healthy and happy.

Brock was having a "guys" weekend. He and a group of racing comrades were at our second home in the Thousand Islands. They would be off to the auto races outside Montreal. Our Christmas Shoppe in the village would be filled with summer travelers.

Then came the call that changed our lives forever.

TWO

"MOM, THEY SAY I HAVE CANCER."

Brock must have driven like a madman to get there in time, but I knew he'd make it to the airport to see me off. I had been running on pure adrenalin for hours—struggling with having to wait for a flight to Los Angeles and not wanting to go at all. I had left my mother, father, and daughter in emotional chaos, but had to resist comforting them and set my mind on the journey ahead. No time for emotions—just that moment in time. Brock hugged me so hard my breath left my body for a moment. He had many questions about Sean, but I had few or no answers to give. We uttered some halting, inadequate words and held each other tight.

As I ran for the airline gate in Rochester and breathlessly boarded the flight for Los Angeles, I felt a sinking feeling in the pit of my stomach that my life would never be the same. From the moment that I heard Sean's words the day before, my orderly world started spinning out of control.

"Mom, I'm in the emergency room in Tarzana Hospital. I hemorrhaged and got myself into a cab. Mom, they say I have cancer. Mom, I'm sorry. Mom, it's not my back. Mom, I'm sorry." How it rolled around in my head like a lyric of a song that you can't forget. I'm ashamed to think that he felt he had to apologize for having cancer or for bothering me.

It wasn't his back. It wasn't a disc problem. All those months, all that pain. My mind raced to sort the emotion from the facts. How could this be happening? What had gone wrong?

Waiting for that morning flight had taken all the self-control I could muster. Within moments a peaceful, pastoral scene was shattered and my whole life, the life of my whole family, had been turned upside down. My sense of peace from knowing my children were all embarking on successful lives—the comfortable scenarios most parents take for granted—gone in a flash. Those years of nurturing Sean, helping him to believe in himself, now gone. All was meaningless in the light of his illness.

Mid-flight, a pilot deadheading home struck up a conversation with me. I didn't want to talk, but he drew me out. Maybe it was a relief not to have to think about our situation. I was okay until he asked the usual perfunctory questions. "What do you do? Do you have children?"

I struggled with my answers. It was the first time I'd have to say it out loud to a stranger. How do I even phrase it? I'd better learn; I'll have to say it from here on out. "I have a daughter in college getting her masters in English literature and, well, until yesterday, uh—you see, my son, he was just starting his life and career in TV production and … ." Breaking down, sobbing the words, "You'll have to excuse me. He was just diagnosed with cancer."

The pilot offered words of encouragement. I thanked him. We were quiet for the rest of the flight.

I had to keep my wits about me. I couldn't show anyone how frightened I was. My stepson, Brock, Jr., had agreed to meet my flight. He is such a dear young man, relaxed, affable, and always there for someone in need. A child of the 1960s, he had moved to Redondo Beach several years before to work at the Portofino Inn, one of the only hotels directly on the ocean. Brocker was born in San Diego when his father was stationed there as a naval officer. The laid-back southern California lifestyle suited him just fine. He met the plane at LAX and delivered me to the hospital.

I wished someone else could have taken me. He'd been through his own hell, as had his sister Claire and brother Dan, after their mother's terrible auto accident some years before, which ultimately led to her death. They'd earned my undying respect for the way they cared for her. Brocker had tried to help and comfort Sean when he was experiencing his excruciating back pain. No one—not even the doctors—knew that it wasn't ordinary pain.

On the way up the 405 freeway I talked to Brocker about everything and anything. There was a desperation in my stream-of-consciousness chatter. From gay, to almost euphoric, and then into the depths of depression. We arrived at the hospital in Tarzana, and I was terrified. I put on my "Mom" mask and, with Brocker at my side, entered the hospital, dreading the reunion. First I had to meet with the doctor who had seen Sean in the emergency room the day before. After a thorough examination, he had diagnosed Sean's cancer. A simple rectal exam revealed a large mass around his prostate. I wanted to talk to the doctor and hear for myself about what he had found. I had to see his body language and expressions when he relayed the information that would affect my son's life and the future of our family. Maybe he had made a horrible mistake. Maybe it was the wrong patient.

While waiting for the doctor I called Brock to let him know I had arrived. Just then a slender, dapper man appeared around the corner. From the nurse's description I knew it was Sean's doctor. I told Brock I would call him later and hung up. Sean's doctor was in his early fifties and looked like a model for GQ. This was the gastroenterologist who had seen Sean in the emergency room. He put out his hand. Slowly I walked toward him, not sure I wanted to connect with him and validate what I was going to hear. He placed his hands on my shoulders as he told me that Sean had a large mass around his prostate. He suspected it was serious, but they wouldn't know until they ran more tests. I swooned and he held me gently while I caught my composure. He also suspected problems in

Sean's abdomen. He was circumspect, but everything he was saying and the way he was saying it made me think Sean was in grave danger.

Sean had to be put through more tests: MRI, bone scan, and gastrointestinal tests. He was in a great deal of pain. It seemed terrible to put him through all that. I rejoined Brocker and relayed the information the doctor had given me. I could see that Brocker was shaken by the news. The look we exchanged spoke volumes. It was time to see Sean. As we approached his room, I wanted to bolt and run. Thankfully, Brocker was with me because I was trying desperately to be brave for both him and Sean. When we reached the door to Sean's room, I grabbed Brocker's hand and we entered together.

I had to stifle a gasp when I saw Sean in the hospital bed. My 6-foot-tall, handsome, sandy-blond-haired boy with sparkling blue eyes and open warm smile had melted into a skinny, gaunt, dead-eyed young man. The change was shocking, but this was now my son. I strode up to Sean, smiling, as if I had just seen him an hour ago and threw my arms around him, or what was left of him.

I backed away as Brocker approached his bedside. Although he was terribly uneasy, he did his best to treat Sean as if he had just had minor surgery. After about ten minutes of awkward small talk, Brocker had to leave. I walked him to the exit. Along the way we never said a word. A big hug, and he was off. How I wished I could escape, too. I was on my own until my husband arrived the next morning.

As I reentered Sean's room, he put his arms out. I ran to him and held him for what seemed an eternity. Sean broke the moment. Out of nowhere, he began to chuckle.

I pulled away and said, "What are you laughing about?"

"Mom, this place is nuts."

As I returned to the chair by his bedside, I was so relieved that he had changed the terrible moment.

"Okay, how so?" I asked.

"There have been so many nurses and doctors in an out of my room that I'm going crazy. I am so tired and they won't give me time to sleep."

I laughed, "You know what they say. If you want to recuperate don't go to a hospital." He smiled weakly, laying his head back on the pillow. Chuckling again. "What now?" I asked. He opened his eyes.

"This is totally not PC but this one doctor came in to see me. He was from Pakistan or India, I don't know, but I couldn't understand a word he said. All I know is that when he asked me where I was from and I told him near Buffalo, New York, he went nuts. All he could say was 'Niagara Falls! Niagara Falls!' It was like a *Three Stooges* routine. I tried to ask him more about my condition, but all he wanted to talk about was Niagara Falls. He left abruptly and that was that. I don't even know what kind of doctor he was."

I was more disturbed than amused about the doctor not answering Sean's concerns. Within seconds, the door swung open and in walked the mysterious doctor Sean had just described. He introduced himself, but he was talking so fast I couldn't understand a word he said. He checked Sean's chart, took his vital signs, then turned to me. "Tell me about Niagara Falls. Is it worth seeing?"

I was caught off guard and reflexively responded. "Ah, well sure it's big. Ah. Sean. What … "

Before I could gain my composure he was out the door. "I will be back," he said as he abruptly exited.

Sean looked at me and I looked at him. We both broke into laughter as Sean shrugged his shoulders and said, "See, I told you so."

Sean's medical team would soon be joined by the doctor in charge of oncology. It was all coming so fast; my mind was overloaded. I couldn't imagine how Sean was dealing with it all.

If the gastroenterologist was a model for *GQ*, the oncologist belonged on the front cover. Fiftyish and wonderfully tanned, wearing a light tan suit with a perfectly matching tie, he walked with a proud gait and beamed a broad smile at us. He seemed to be warmly welcomed and respected by all who came in contact with him. I mused that even doctors in Los Angeles looked like actors. Was it a prerequisite for getting a job?

Sean's pain was being handled well, probably for the first time in months. I think he was so glad to be safe and have me near that it dwarfed the reality of the situation. He had been dealing with his sickness by himself for so long it had become a way of life. He seemed resigned to whatever had to be done to him. I could see how his suffering had altered his personality. Sean had always resisted going to the doctor and, frankly, I seldom ever knew he was ill.

I watched him drift off to sleep. The combination of the medication and the doctor's information exhausted him. I suspected his sleeping was also a means of escape. Sean was all alone when he first learned about his cancer. I was haunted by the thought that he had been suffering alone.

"Mom." I was startled out of my reverie by the tone in Sean's voice. He anxiously asked me to call his orthopedic surgeon. "Tell him what's happened; tell him I have cancer. That I'm really sick."

I couldn't get used to hearing those words—I didn't ever want to hear them. The most incredible thing was that Sean wanted to prove to the doctor who performed his spinal surgery that he hadn't been faking his pain. How horribly sad it made me to think that he felt the need at that time to convince that doctor of the authenticity of his illness. How could this highly recommended orthopedic surgeon witness a vigorous young man's rapid decline and obvious pain and never order a complete physical? A simple rectal exam or an examination of Sean's abdomen might have revealed the real cause months ago.

How could a professional have been so narrowly focused as to miss such a diagnosis? Sean surmised that the doctor thought he was simply looking for pain pills. You would think that after Sean lost forty-five pounds, someone, especially his doctor, would have looked further for the truth.

As Sean drifted off again, I couldn't stop thinking about the orthopedist and how he had misdiagnosed Sean's condition. And then the real torment began: Why hadn't *we* done more during those last months? I should have known there was something more serious than a spinal disc problem after his surgery. But I allowed myself to believe that Sean was in the hands of a well known specialist. I'd checked his credentials and kept in close touch. I thought I had been an advocate. But the doctor wasn't concerned about more than back problems. Certainly no one suspected a serious illness.

I staggered down the hall to the pay phone, my only lifeline to the outside world.

As I reached the phone, my rage was building. I was ready to call Sean's physician and confront him. How would he respond to the news? Could he explain his mistakes?

At first, I panicked and couldn't remember the phone number. Then, after what seemed an eternity, the doctor's assistant answered. I asked to speak with the doctor, but she told me he was busy with patients and would get back to me. I told her that Sean was in the hospital. She became quiet, understanding my tone. "Tell the doctor he'd better get on the phone. Sean has cancer." Dead air, then, "Hold on, I'll get him."

A moment later the doctor was on the line: "Mrs. Yates?"

"Yes" I replied.

"What's going on? Sean has cancer? How could that be? What happened?"

I blurted out, "How could you have been caring for him and not notice?"

Silence.

"Where did they find the cancer?"

I told him all the information I knew at that point.

He said his wife was an oncology nurse at UCLA Medical Center and then gave me his private cell phone number. "Please call me anytime," he insisted.

It used to always take dozens of steps to reach him. Now, wonder of wonders, I got his private line and could call anytime. He also told me to forget his bill.

He sounded off balance, shaken, and a little nervous. He should have been.

By mid-afternoon, my cousin, Roberta, arrived. She was the daughter of Edith, one of my mother's four sisters. Edith had been ill for years and died at thirty-five, leaving a husband and three teenage daughters. My mother had cared for Edith, as she had her other siblings, in her final days. Cancer had taken all of them—Betty, Gus, Edith, and Joe.

I remember going with my mother to visit my Aunt Edith when I was five years old. She lived in a walk-up apartment in the Bronx. I was drawn to Edith's long fingernails which she kept beautifully manicured. They were her one source of pride. I would sit for hours putting on my Aunt Edith's makeup while my mother cooked for her and greeted the girls when they arrived home from school. The most memorable of my visits involved a pair of scissors and Aunt Edith's curtains. My mother had been teaching me to cut out paper dolls. Sitting in the open window against the fire escape, I was shredding the curtains when my mother spotted me. She was horrified, but Aunt Edith dissolved into laughter. As my mother scolded me, Roberta arrived home from school and witnessed the mayhem. She quickly grabbed me, consoled my mother, and took me to the local movie theatre. She instantly became my hero. Not too long after that episode, Aunt Edith passed away. The girls were devastated. Roberta was inconsolable; she drove off to California to seek her fortune. In the 1950s that was a big deal. She learned the skill of art film color stripping and became one of the best in the business.

I hadn't seen her since Sean's back surgery in May. Thankfully, she was close to him and kept in touch. Roberta had expressed her frustration many times that Sean seemed to be avoiding her. Now we all finally realized why. Living with his pain had become his life. He resisted seeing people because it put pressure on him to get involved, and his pain-ridden body couldn't handle it. He was tired and embarrassed at having to make excuses for himself.

Roberta and her son David had cleaned up Sean's apartment after he hemorrhaged and was rushed to the hospital. She had become a very religious person. It felt good to have her with me to help pass the time and provide comfort. When at last she had to leave for work, she gave me her house key and said that her home was open to us for as long as we needed it.

That day seemed endless. When Sean was awake we talked—short bursts of conversation, questions from him about his condition, many of which I couldn't answer. He spoke by phone with Alex, a good friend from his prep school days, who was living in Boston. Alex had survived testicular cancer and was now doing fine. Sean took comfort from him. Alex was someone his own age who had been there and knew.

I wasn't as comforted. We weren't dealing with the same disease. But I couldn't let Sean know my misgivings. It would spoil his hopes and reinforce his fears.

A moment of levity occurred when Sean overheard a nurse commenting on how young his mother looked. "Mom, they say you look more like my wife than my mother." He seemed genuinely amused by this. I kidded him, too, but secretly knew that if the cancer hadn't altered his looks and aged him so, they never would have thought that. As long as he was amused, it was okay.

Sean drifted in and out of sleep, assisted by painkillers. While he slept, I called my husband. Brock would have to carry a heavy burden at home while loving us and helping us fight our war. Early that evening he arrived at the hospital. I tried to soften the blow but, of course, it was no use. This could not be downplayed.

I filled Brock in on what had been discussed so far. We met a few doctors who would perform the tests the next morning. They already told Sean that he had to drink a gallon of a vile liquid called "Go Lightly." The awful-tasting stuff had to be taken every two hours during the night until the entire gallon was gone. This process would cleanse his system so that they could perform a colonoscopy to determine if the cancer had spread. After that would come major abdominal surgery. Information was pouring in from all over. Family and friends were networking like crazy. It's amazing how many people have suffered the great equalizers—illness and death.

By the third day Sean's pain seemed to be under control and he was not sleeping as much. The hospital oncology library was inundating him with literature on cancer. Books arrived. The most well known were, *When Bad Things Happen to Good People* and *The Power of Positive Thinking*. He was reading like mad, desperately trying to come to terms with what was happening to him, looking for magical insight that would reinforce his hope.

He'd always shied away from seeking help. I could never even get him into counseling after his father and I divorced. He always turned everything inward.

Now he had to reach out.

Four days had passed since my arrival and rarely had I seen Sean smile. Then his friend Dennis arrived with a picture that his daughter Zoe had colored for Sean. She was only four and had a crush on Sean. According to Dennis, when Zoe visited the office Sean would hide under his desk, playing hide and seek with her even when suffering with his back pain. He carried her picture in his wallet.

I was constantly amazed at how tender Sean was with little children. He had always cried easily when he was a boy and took such heat for it from the other kids. If there was an injured bird, Sean would bring it home. I often felt life might have been easier for him if he hadn't been so sensitive.

I remember going through the hospital lobby and seeing a man who passed me carrying a big stuffed teddy bear sporting a blue bow. He was on his way to celebrate a new life, a little boy. What a contrast between us, I thought, with our son desperately ill on the next floor.

A hospital is a strange place, a place where a new life enters the world as another life exits. It was hard to get my mind around that. Nights were hard. I had to leave Sean in the hospital each evening after the crush of the day's events, the deluge of information, the penetrating pain, and the inability to process the grief. In bed at night, the realities of Sean's illness filled my head with a deafening roar. I couldn't clear my mind, let alone sleep. How could I put my heart and mind on hold? How could I get enough rest to meet the next day? The next reality? I'd never fully appreciated the blessing of sleep. Would I ever again? On the fourth night, the eve of Sean's exploratory surgery, we didn't sleep at all. I just lay in Brock's arms crying. Not really crying, actually, almost whimpering, like a wounded animal caught in a trap.

Sean's surgery was scheduled for 8:00 a.m. Brock and I got up in plenty of time to fight the freeway traffic and make sure we were there to kiss him and be some comfort before his surgery. We were terrified. Thankfully, he didn't know this surgery would determine where the cancer originated and just how far it had spread. He was too sick and uncomfortable to sort out the information, let alone his emotions. It had all come so fast we'd had no time to process it.

We arrived on Sean's floor and walked the long corridor toward his room, stopping just before the doorway to muster our positive energy before having to face him. We entered the room. Something was wrong! His room was empty. Not only empty, but dark and lifeless. I shrieked and bolted, rushing past doorway after doorway. Wild, horrible thoughts flooded my mind. I thought he had died and I hadn't been there for him. Reaching the nurses' station, I could barely gasp the question, "Sean Reynolds?"

One of the nurses grabbed me, seeing how frantic I was. I spun around and confronted her.

"Sean Reynolds. What happened to him? Where is he? Is he dead?" I sobbed.

She turned to another nurse. "Sean Reynolds. Where is he?"

Another nurse spoke up, "He's gone to surgery."

"Surgery? It can't be, I told him we'd be here! When? Take me to him now! He can't be alone, not my baby, he's so scared." Brock and I bolted down the corridor, both of us frantic. The nurses ran after us and blocked our way. They said we couldn't see him. The surgery had been pushed up.

I began crying and pleading. "What if he dies without knowing we were here? What if I never get to tell him I love him?"

I couldn't remember much for the next few minutes, except that we found ourselves with my cousin Roberta, who had arrived by then. I was sitting in a waiting room thumbing through the Book of Psalms, reading the same passages over and over. If I could say them fervently enough and often enough, perhaps it would all go away and I'd wake up from the nightmare.

Several hours went by and then a call came. Sean was out of surgery. They told us it had been an incredibly complicated surgery, but he was okay. The doctor would meet us in the main hospital waiting room. I remember that I was almost more upset that the surgery was over because now we would have to confront the findings. Neither of us said a word as we headed for the waiting room. Each of us was overwhelmed with emotions and possibilities unimaginable only days earlier.

Brock took my hand. I was thinking, what a civilized culture we live in. No one passing us would have suspected we were on our way to learn if our son was going to live or die. There's an etiquette to everything—be stoic, don't embarrass yourselves, keep a stiff upper lip. Then we were in the waiting room and moments later the doctor was sitting next to us. Trying to size him up, I wondered, does he look like it's good news or bad news? I couldn't get a reading.

They did this everyday. I couldn't even imagine choosing this for a career. Our child—to him just a patient. I guess that's how it must be or he couldn't get through it.

"Well, we found the primary; sometimes you never know where it starts. It's adeno-carcinoma appendicle."

"You mean his appendix?" I asked.

"Yes, it's rare, maybe only three hundred fifty people we know of. We debulked about two pounds of tumor."

Neither Brock nor I could look at one another. Brock said, "Well, if you've found out where it originated, isn't that good? Can't you get it all?"

I knew instantly by the doctor's face it wouldn't be that way. My brain had already processed the information and jumped to what I instinctively knew was the prognosis.

"No, it doesn't matter in this kind of cancer because it's mucous spreading. It travels easily and spreads almost like a slime and surrounds everything."

I said, " What about multiple surgeries to clean it out?"

"It's been done along with chemo, but it hasn't been very successful and, frankly, it's terribly painful and hard on the patients."

"When can we see him?"

"Give him a few hours and then he'll be in ICU overnight until he stabilizes."

We thanked him. I couldn't help thinking, again, how civilized we were. Why would you thank someone for that? It is puzzling how we just blindly go through the motions, never really analyzing why we say and do the things we do. It's all so reflexive and empty. Why didn't I scream and cry and rip my hair out?

In the United States—I can only speak for the people I know—we often look down on people of other cultures, who wail and pull out their hair when a loved one dies. Maybe their way isn't so awful or strange; it may be raw and hard to witness, but at least it's honest.

Hours passed as Brock, Roberta, Sean's various friends and coworkers, and I kept vigil. Each was lost in his or her own thoughts and memories. We were all searching our emotions and wondering how we would face Sean again. What would we say to him?

The call came that Sean was in the ICU and Brock and I could see him briefly. As we passed a window, I realized it was evening. A whole day had passed while we were immersed in this ordeal. We walked briskly, but neither of us wanted to see him—not there, not knowing what we knew.

We left Roberta in the small ICU waiting room. I headed through the double doors into a little unit of high tech and silence where lives are held in precarious balance. A nurse led us to Sean's room. Looking in, we saw two nurses standing over a bed performing their tasks efficiently and with great speed. As one of them moved away, I realized the person lying there was Sean. In the half-light, I could make out his face, and by the movement of his body, I could tell he was suffering. I moved in closer as if walking on eggshells. I approached his bed just as he was turning his head toward the door. There in the dim light my child lay desperately ill. All I could see were his eyes wide with fear and pain, a haunting sight, imploring me. He could not speak but his eyes said volumes. *Mom, I'm so glad to see you. Mom, this is dreadful. Mom, I hurt so much. Mom, no one told me it would be so bad. Mom, help me!*

Tears rolled down my face as I made a feeble attempt to smile. The nurses ushered me out so that they could get his pain under control and make him more comfortable.

I stood in the hallway, looking back at him in the half-light of that grim setting. He never took his eyes off me. I'll never forget it for as long as I live, those eyes, large as saucers, hollow, penetrating, imploring me.

I could do nothing. No torture could be greater. He was all alone, even with us present.

Brock dragged me out the doors. I felt a pressure in my chest and everything started to spin out of control. I started to pull for air; I swooned and Roberta and Brock caught me and got me to a chair. All I could say was, "My baby. It should have been me in there."

A bitter struggle began in me as I debated whether we should tell Sean the whole ugly truth. I knew Brock's feelings. He was the eternal optimist. He would never give up hope, nor did he think Sean should. But I'd seen too much cancer in my family not to know what the future held. The current wisdom is to tell the patient everything. Each of us must deal with our own mortality from a different place. Old people integrate it differently from how the young process it. Where do hope and courage come from? Sean was always such a lonely person, so willing to turn inward and blame himself. How could we take the chance he would give up? How could I rob him of even more precious time? How could I bear to watch my son learn that he was going to die?

Here is my advice to you: *Don't let conventional wisdom dictate your decision.*

You know your loved one. You have the right to decide whether he or she will benefit or not from knowing the truth.

The death of a young person is a very different thing from the death of an old person.

Factor in the reasons for full disclosure, but use your best judgment and stand your ground.

THREE

LEAVING LOS ANGELES

I drove with Brock to the doctor's office on a beautiful California day. If I had closed my mind to the past days of hospitals and sickness, we could have been heading out to see friends for lunch. There was so much to say and think about, yet somehow the words were far away. All alone, we were surrounded by deafening silence.

The doctor's office was in one of those endlessly ordinary office buildings—yet inside waited a man with news far from ordinary. News so important that it would dictate the rest of our son's life.

We waited in a small, tastefully decorated waiting room for what seemed an eternity, surrounded by many people in different stages of illness. It was a world-in-miniature, filled with heart-wrenching stories.

Finally a nurse showed us into the doctor's office. The walls were covered with pictures of family, photo ops at fund-raisers with celebrities, and medical degrees. I moved from photo to photo trying to put together a sense of this man who held the life of my child in his hands.

The silence was broken as Dr. Bluming entered and greeted us with an open smile. Speaking in soft, warm tones with plenty of eye contact, he radiated humanity. There was initially some small talk, then I asked, "How can you do what you do? Where do you bury the sadness?" My thoughts were spilling out. There was no time for patience.

He said that, when he first became an oncologist twenty years before, he had a partner and they specialized in pediatric cancer. Ninety percent of their patients died. His partner committed suicide. He told us that now he deals with all types of cancer, and the survival rates had dramatically improved. It was in the hope of survival that he found his strength.

I blurted out, "Sean must *not* know he is terminal."

The doctor took a deep breath, "He is an emancipated male, of legal age, and in that case we always tell the patient."

"I don't care. I don't want him to know. He may be emancipated in the eyes of the law, but he is *my* child, and *I* know him best. For the most part he views life in a negative light. I don't want him to retreat to his bed and dwell on dying. He has been robbed of enough time already."

Reluctantly, the doctor agreed. Sean would not find out through him. He said he respected my decision, and said, "I cannot imagine what I would do if it were my child."

Breaking the awkward moment, Brock asked, "When does chemo begin and what will the side effects be? When can he leave the hospital? Will he be strong enough to travel?"

My mind was racing ahead. All I wanted to know was the bottom line. I asked, "How will it be? What will his death be like?"

Brock seemed startled, twisting in his chair. I realized he hadn't let his mind go there yet. While I was sorry to disorient him, it was something I had to know. I couldn't bear it anymore. We needed to be prepared for what seemed to be inevitable.

The doctor became quiet and paused as he looked at me. "Wow." he said, . "*You* are asking the *hard* questions." He struggled to answer.

His body language told me Sean's last days were going to be dreadful. Tears welled up in my eyes as I struggled to keep my composure. "I *have* to know. You must understand."

He looked stoically at me and said, "Hard, very hard."

After that, I remember nothing of the meeting. My mind and heart felt numb. I couldn't even cry.

As we left the doctor's office, Brock turned and took me in his arms, kissing me gently on the forehead. I buried my face in his chest as the tears flowed. We held on to each other tightly, both lost in our own realities as we tried to find some comfort. We were feeling hopelessly vulnerable.

As we drove away, Brock gave me the details I had missed. He said Sean would be hooked up to a chemo pump that he could carry around—a new technique. As his pain increased, morphine could be added to the chemo. He would need another small operation to run the IV lines into his chest and from there to his arteries. The access lines, or Hickman catheter, would come out of the top of his chest. It's much easier and less painful to administer medications through these lines than through subcutaneous shots. Small blessing, I guessed.

Outside, the sun was still shining. People hustled and bustled with what seemed to me not a care in the world. How could everyone act so carefree when my world was crumbling?

The endless ooze of concrete buildings and parking lots covered with graffiti and ugly signage depressed me. The lack of skyscrapers in L.A. results in miles of urban sprawl. Everything looks the same. After driving for sometime I saw a beautiful Spanish-style Catholic church—its arbors covered with lush vines and crimson flowers. The expanse of lawns and old stone walking paths drew me in. This touch of old world tranquility sandwiched in between the modern, cold architecture was representative of the cultural blend of new Los Angles. It was striking. I hadn't been to church in years. Now I was feeling the need to sit inside a church in the presence of mysteries and powers greater than my small universe.

Often Brock and I were asked about our faith. We would always respond that we were "spiritual"—a common cliché. Brock was not raised in a home with a disciplined religious tradition. He found God in his everyday world, constantly appreciating the great gifts of life, such as the beauty of the environment and the natural laws that govern life. He believed that the universe and life must be governed by a higher power. These were beliefs we shared.

My religious experiences had been different. I was raised a Catholic. My father was Italian and my mother a Jew. I loved to hear my mother's father tell the story about how he used to chase after my father with a baseball bat yelling, "I have nothing against you personally, but stay away from my daughter. A mixed faith marriage won't work."

My father and my grandfather ultimately became fast friends. Mom and Dad were married by a justice of the peace, and my mother agreed to raise me in the Catholic faith. Even as a young girl of nine or ten, I felt close to God. Doing good works, both then and now, was a big part of my life. Yet my father did not practice his faith. Ironically, my Jewish mother was the most Christ-like person I knew. Her goodness and love were the compass I used to guide my journey through life.

If it hadn't been for an old Italian priest in a small Catholic church in White Plains, New York, where I grew up, I might have stayed in the church. He knew my parents had not been married in the Catholic church and, when I was twelve years old, took me aside and told me I was illegitimate. Then he pleaded with me to go home and convince my parents to get married in the church to establish my legitimacy. His comment wounded me deeply. Luckily, I was mature for my age and well grounded—believing my God would never judge in that way. It wasn't until years later that I shared this with my parents. I knew that if I had told my father about it, being the hot-headed Italian that he was, he would most likely have gone to the church and punched the priest.

After that I turned away from organized religion, believing my faith and strength came from God. I strived to be the best person I could. To me a successful and godly life comes from the way we connect to our fellow humans, forming a chain of positive energy that can be felt, shared, and passed on.

When I spotted the church that day I asked Brock to park the car. Without saying a word I bolted down the old brick stones leading to the church entrance. It looked more like a Spanish mission than the Catholic churches I knew on the East Coast. The huge, old, dark wooden doors were intimidating, but the need to find some inner peace drove me past my fears. As I reached the giant doorknobs, I felt Brock's hand touch mine. We exchanged loving smiles and entered the church. It was like going back to my childhood. I approached a cluster of wrought iron stands containing candles. Many of them were already lit, telling me I was not alone. Each candle represented another soul searching for some comfort. I lit a candle, made the sign of the cross, and dropped to my knees. All the pressure, the fear, the sorrow, and the pain came to the surface. I began to cry, and asked, "God, why have you forsaken us? Help me to find the strength and love to be what my son and family need. Be with me so I can handle this dreadful situation." I felt a hand on my shoulder. It was the priest. His face was heavily lined and his balding head had errant wisps of gray hair scattered over it. Hearing me weeping, he had come to sit with me. After a few moments he whispered, "My daughter, be not afraid." His presence calmed me.

I wondered how long Sean and I would have together. How many more days and nights would we share until he was gone? No matter how hard you may try to deny it, the human spirit, I am convinced, needs to believe in a supreme power. Why else would our minds and souls have wrapped themselves around the concept? It's been a part of our consciousness since the earliest recorded history. What's the expression? "More than we know. More than we can ever know."

That evening we had dinner with John and Cathy Mullin, dear friends and Sean's boss and mentor in the television industry. Their love for us and kindness toward Sean had been a source of comfort for us all. Sean's love and respect for John was touching because he didn't get close to many people. He often told me, "You know Mom, sometimes I believe John thinks of me as a son." It seemed to make Sean happy. He obviously looked to John for approval and was gratified by his friendship and mentoring.

All the conversation revolved around Sean and the months to come. It was horrific to talk that way about Sean—his illness, and the future, such as it was. After a pregnant pause, John approached the subject of having Sean meet with a psychologist, somehing that had never entered my mind. Brock and I agreed it might be a good idea, but Sean, being very private, would be hard to convince if he didn't see the merits.

John recommended a psychologist he trusted, someone in his mid-thirties. John said he had known him for years and thought Sean would like him. We all agreed that Sean would benefit from talking with someone—and soon. My job would be to convince him.

After three days Sean's abdominal pain was at a tolerable level and his spirits were upbeat. While the long-term realities remained the same, whenever Sean felt better we considered it a gift.

Brock had been holding off but was under pressure from *Car and Driver* magazine to complete an assignment. It was an interview with Jay Leno, a long-time friend and fellow car nut. Jay had an eclectic collection of interesting toys, cars, and motorcycles. What is so wonderful about Jay is that, unlike many people with fame, he used and enjoyed his toys. They didn't just sit in some garage gathering dust. Brock asked me to come along since it was such a beautiful day and we needed to get away from the hospital for a while.

"I think you'll enjoy meeting Jay. He's a great guy." Brock promised.

We asked Sean if we could leave him for a little while. He said, "Gosh, why wouldn't you? It's work. Go ahead; I'll be okay. Jay Leno is one of my heroes. Wish I could go along. Tell him I'm a big fan."

Heading down the freeways to L.A. I was reminded how heavily traveled the roads were. Sean always said that no one travels too far, too often. After living in western New York, where the roads were open and free of traffic, our patience was tested. But, still, it felt good to be away from the hospital for a short time.

When we arrived at Jay Leno's garage he came to the door to greet us. I felt like a fan sizing him up to see if he looked the same in person as on TV. I held out my hand and, with his warm smile, he put me immediately at ease. He was sweet, shy, unaffected—just another car guy like hundreds I'd met with Brock over the years. It's always so interesting how the "car thing" is a great equalizer. Rich or poor—around cars, everyone is the same.

I followed Brock and Jay around like a puppy as they strolled through his museum/workshop. His collection was impressive. I counted about fifty vehicles of various shapes and sizes, all with different kinds of power sources. Jay is a hands-on collector, working alongside his team of full-time restorationists.

Jay took us from one vehicle to another explaining, in excruciating detail, how each worked. I say "excruciating" because my personal knowledge of automobiles could be put in a tiny thimble, even though I am married to one of the world's leading automotive journalists. Jay asked me if I remembered learning about internal combustion in chemistry class in school. I laughed out loud and told him I couldn't even remember taking chemistry in school, let alone remember anything about internal combustion!

It was a fascinating afternoon. Both Jay and Brock talked nonstop. I wanted to laugh out loud because it all sounded like a foreign language to me. I did get caught up in their enthusiasm, however, and found myself really looking at the cars and motorcycles from a different perspective.

Jay had heard about Sean's condition and expressed his regrets. Realizing how awkward Jay felt, I quickly told him that Sean was a great fan of his. Without pause he said, "Well, let's call him up and say hello." Within minutes he was talking to Sean. He said, "Sean this is Jay Leno. How are you doing, Buddy?" It was a fantastic gesture from a wonderful guy.

We couldn't wait to get back to the hospital to hear Sean's reaction. As we passed the nurses' station everyone was smiling. One called out, "Sean is a happy man today."

When we entered Sean's room he said, "Mom! Brock! Do you know who called me?" Before we could respond he said, "I felt like an idiot. I thought it was one of the guys playing a joke. But it was really him. Wow, he was so nice. He told me to get well and get out of bed."

We laughed. "We know, we know, we were right there. He just picked up the phone when we told him you were recovering from surgery. Great guy, huh?" Sean's smile said it all.

Great guy indeed! Jay will never realize how much his kind gesture lifted Sean's spirits.

The day came for Sean's next surgery. Putting a Hickman line in Sean's chest would be a short, mercifully simple process. Sean was ready and willing to get the surgery over, confident that the wisdom of the experts and his full cooperation would speed up his ultimate recovery. Like so many of the medical steps we were to take in the future, we had no idea of the repercussions and emotions that would come. The surgery went off without any difficulty. When Sean got back to his room he was awake and in good spirits. He was told that chemo could begin the next day, and he could be released the day after.

"Well Mom," Sean said, "the worst is past. Soon I can rejoin the guys at *Truckin' USA*. They're holding my job."

Brock bounced back quickly, "I spoke with John Coleman yesterday, and he said the crew is looking forward to going for shwarma, but they won't touch a bite until you return."

"I sure love that stuff. I never thought I would get to love exotic Middle Eastern food when I left little Wyoming, New York," Sean said, smiling.

Brock and I left Sean that day feeling relieved that he would soon be out of the hospital and in our care. After all, leaving the hospital is traditionally a sign that one is getting better.

The next day we saw that Sean's mood was improving as his pain was finally being handled properly. It was a revelation to see the difference that pain management could make in a person who was so ill. It was time for me to open the discussion about the need for him to talk with a psychologist. I struggled with the right words to say if he resisted. After my divorce, I had tried to get him to go for therapy. He refused, saying he could handle it by himself. It was a typical response, especially from an 11-year-old boy with low self-esteem. He could never admit to not being able to handle a situation.

"Sean, I think you need to talk to someone not emotionally involved in your illness. You have been through so much and will be going through so much more. It might be helpful."

He paused briefly, reflecting on what I had just said and then responded, "Okay Mom, can you help me find someone?"

I was stunned. I left that day realizing how important it is to find ways to provide hope to those facing illness.

The next day we prepared Roberta's spare bedroom for Sean's homecoming. It was small, but comfy and cheerful. We were very nervous about taking him out of the hospital. Now he was in our care, and I was terrified. How could I cope with a son who was terminally ill? With only a few minutes of instruction I was still unsure how to work the chemo pump. Sean would be totally dependent on me for his comfort. I couldn't reveal my trepidation—it was time to put on a happy face.

Brock and I arrived at the hospital cheering each other up almost as if we were in a pep rally. We were ready for Sean's homecoming. Brock told stories of people he knew who had survived terrible illnesses. I, too, had heard of such stories—

hopeful stories for two parents who were frightened to face the future. As we approached Sean's room Brock squeezed my hand. The room was dark and we could barely see Sean, who lay in a fetal position on his side. He did not acknowledge our presence. What had happened since yesterday? How could they possibly think he could go home today?

I frantically ran to the nurses' station, "How can we take him home like this. What happened to him?"

The nurse put her arms around me and held me. The tears and fear came flooding out. I was stripped clean of pretense. As she held me, she said that, sometimes, when the chemo begins, a combination of reality and chemicals make the patients regress for a time. She assured me it would be temporary and he would soon be okay.

No one had prepared us for this. We called the doctor, who said we should wait until Sean felt well enough to leave the hospital.

By the end of the day Sean began to respond. At one point he said, "Mom, I am frightened about the chemo. It feels so weird, I'm embarrassed to walk around with this stuff in me."

Later that day we took him home from the hospital. He was now in our care.

The first night I looked in on Sean a dozen times. He was restless, and I didn't know what to do for him. His body was getting used to the chemo pump, his constant companion. I know he was a little frightened to be away from the security of the hospital with his new equipment.

I barely slept at all; I kept listening for him.

Half dreaming, I heard, *beep, beep, beep.* Then a plaintive wail.

"Mom! Brock!"

"Oh my God! Brock, the pump."

"What pump?"

I shook Brock. "Sean's calling." Instantly, I realized what must have happened, and we rushed into Sean's room.

"Mom, my pump is beeping. It's out. I pulled it out. I didn't mean to."

"It's okay, honey. It's okay." Brock called the doctor. Suddenly, we were in the car heading to the doctor's office. The thing wouldn't stop beeping. We were all trying to stay calm. When we got to Dr. Bluming's office, they immediately got us into one of the examination rooms. The pump was quickly and easily reconnected. Still scared, but relieved, we stayed there in silence for half an hour. Then we returned to our temporary home. Our lives were now totally in the hands of medical science.

I started a nightly journal, but writing in it was so painful, I debated the effort. However, I was becoming aware that it was better to spread my thoughts and emotions out on paper than to struggle with and internalize them. It helped me to keep my sanity during such a terrible time.

Once Sean was safe and tucked away at Roberta's house, it was time to go to his apartment to clean and pack up his life. Roberta took the day off to care for Sean so that Brock and I could be free to do everything necessary to get him home to New York. We tackled the sad task of gathering his possessions for shipment. Sean's apartment had become a dark and dreary place with the smell of sickness and loneliness permeating every nook and corner.

Two of Brock's children, Brocker and Claire, along with Claire's husband, Bobby, came over and helped. The three of them were sharing a house in Redondo Beach. With all their friends dropping in for dinner each night it was more of a commune. Claire loved to cook and Bobby loved to eat. They had not been married long before they moved from Portland, Oregon, to California. Bobby had been promoted and transferred due to his fast-track career at Chrysler Corporation. He was a loveable, affable, young man. All Brock's children get along so well, each watching out for the other. They had tried many times to take Sean under their wings, and he wanted to let them, but his increasing pain always got in the way.

Goblin, Sean's poor, confused little cat was alone without his master. Sean had been ill for so long that the cat wasn't used to people, and it took a lot of coaxing to get the kitty out from under the bed. We finally managed and then we returned to Roberta's with Goblin and finished our preparations for travel. We couldn't wait to get Sean back to Wyoming, but our anticipation was tempered with a heavy dose of dread.

As the plane began its descent into Rochester, I felt my heart sink. We had come full circle. The feelings and fears I had experienced during my departure on that sad flight to L.A. three weeks earlier came flooding back.

Because Sean was so thin and emaciated we wanted to get him a wheelchair at the airport, but he refused. He was sure he could make it on his own. We ended up having to help him off the plane. How would Stacy react when she saw her brother? I had tried to prepare her with descriptions of how Sean looked and what he had been through. But describing it to someone and their actually seeing it are two different things. Brock and I had been with Sean for three weeks, and even though he was almost unrecognizable, we had gotten used to his appearance. He had always been obsessive about his looks, not wanting to go out if his hair wasn't right. Now he walked through the airport too tired and beat up to even care. All he wanted was to be home where he didn't have to be afraid and alone. Homecomings are supposed to be joyous reunions. This one was not.

To Stacy's credit, she met us with an upbeat smile. It was only when she turned around and headed for the parking lot that I saw her begin to sob. For a young person of twenty-three, death is an abstraction, a non-issue. Suddenly, I felt panic, for my son, for us, and now for my daughter. She was about to begin a journey into a reality that would alter the course of her life. Stacy and Sean had never been close, and I wondered how the dynamics of his illness would play out in their relationship during his remaining months. I wanted to protect her, and him, and us. My emotions were all crazy and I kept trying to keep my equilibrium and gain some perspective. Nothing was making any sense.

The bags arrived, jolting me to my senses and the task at hand—getting Sean home. It was a long, quiet ride; one of many to come.

How defeated Sean must have felt, coming home like this, leaving his future behind. I continued to be thankful that he didn't know the truth. It would be unbearable for him. He had to have hope to fight this terrible disease.

As I passed Sean's room, I glanced in and saw that he was helping his shy, junkyard kitty get used to his new surroundings. I heard him tell Goblin how lucky he was to be here in a place like this. A sweet, unforgettable moment. The reality that this junkyard cat would long survive Sean seared into my heart.

As I walked through the house turning out the lights later that evening, I found Sean sitting outside on the front porch overlooking the valley that stretched before us. The moon was full; it was a beautiful, late-summer night. All we could hear was the chatter of the crickets through the darkness.

Sean sat in one of the rocking chairs and took a long drag on his cigarette. I tiptoed out on the porch, trying not to spoil the moment. "Hi honey. Glad to be home?" He replied, "It's so quiet here, Mom, and the air smells good. I missed the stars in California. The smog is horrible. You'll never know how great it feels to be home. I love you, Mom."

Early the next morning, Barbara, our secretary, was on the intercom. The oncologist from the clinic in Buffalo was on the phone. He explained that he had been briefed on our son's case. I told him about Sean's history of back pain and that he had been operated on for a bad disc.

Without a moment's pause, he matter-of-factly stated it

wasn't his back. It was the cancer. I was taken offguard by his icy response.

I squirmed in my seat and forced myself to ask a question, the answer of which I really didn't want to know. Sean's cancer. "Is there any hope?"

Before I could continue, he responded, "No. None."

I felt like I'd been shot. The abruptness and coldness of his statement left me speechless. I fumbled for the words to respond.

I asked about clinical research. "Wasn't there some hope there?" He must have been aware of the fear and desperation in my voice, but there wasn't any humanity on the other end of the line.

We exchanged some further information, but I swear I can't remember anything that came after that cryptic, emphatic "no."

The doctor had pronounced Sean D.O.A. even before seeing him. How could that be? How could we get through the next months without hope?

The regular pilgrimage to the hospital in Buffalo began. One hour each way, Brock and I in the front seat and our sweet, sick boy in the rear.

We vowed we would help Sean keep his hope for as long as we could. How I hated the secret. How fractured our lives had become—this dance between the truth and fiction, life and death.

We drove the hour in almost total silence, each of us grappling with our own realities and fears.

I tried not to think. I employed all my faculties to close the compartments in my brain that exposed me to pain and emotion. It was a skill I had learned at an early age in order to survive my father's alcoholism. Brock was the one I was worried about. He was trying to be strong for each of us when I knew full well he needed a good cry.

Sean and I entered the hospital lobby and started the incredibly banal task of processing the paperwork. I wanted to

scream with fear and rage at the painful impersonality of bureaucracy.

What was Sean feeling? I wanted to grab him, hold him,
rock him, and protect him from this.

The lobby was huge, black and gray, reminding me of
an old black-and-white newsreel. People were walking as if
in slow motion, the land of the living dead—God's waiting
room—each in desperate search of their own miracle. Each
numbed by pain and fear.

We waited and waited in the lobby. One person after another went through the doors. All I could think of was a
deli counter. Take a number please and wait your turn. How
impersonal and lonely. Sean Reynolds—his name was finally
called. I raced ahead of him to handle the formalities.

I did most of the talking. These days I was speaking more
and more for him. He was withdrawing and seemed perfectly
content to let me carry the load. Sean had turned his life over
to me. The doctors were concerned because he didn't ask
many questions about his treatment or illness. After they had
processed Sean's information, we were directed to another
waiting room toward the back of the hospital. This waiting
room was fairly small and crammed with patients and their
families. It was the colon cancer clinic.

In the clinic waiting room no one talked. Denial, fear, iso-
lation—these permeated the air. It was almost as if people
feared the cancer was contagious.

The staff and nurses in the clinic behaved like wardens
in a leper colony. Someone pointed out our doctor. He was
young, tall, slim, and austere looking.

I was determined to catch him before he met with Sean.
He might employ the current wisdom of full disclosure. Not
with *my* son. No way were they going to tell him he's going
to die a horrible death. That is the way we wanted it. I knew
in my heart that's what Sean would want, too. Brock and I
took the doctor aside and firmly stated our case. No full disclosure. He mumbled something about Sean's being an adult.

I was firm and said that may be true, but he was still our son. We reached an agreement, and though the doctor was not happy, it was settled the way we wanted it.

The doctor agreed to continue the more aggressive therapy that was begun in California. I suspected he was just going through the motions. No clever new treatments, no curiosity, no desire to experiment, no clinical trials—so disappointing. A well known cancer institute like this? You would have thought they could offer more. It seemed we could have gotten the same treatment almost anywhere. If you don't have a disease that can advance their protocols, it seems as if they simply flush you through the system. A cynical numbers game.

Our trip to the hospital was a traumatic experience for all of us. With each exposure to a new hospital, doctor, or clinic, the magnitude of Sean's illness and the awesome realities sunk in further. Life was taking on a surreal quality of wild jumble of emotion and uncertainty coupled with the mundane and routine of our day-to-day lives. One of the blessings of that day-to-day life was Dolores—my faithful friend and housekeeper. Being a country woman and used to getting up early to feed the horses, she arrived at our house before dawn. She had been helping me take care of our house for years. Through our ups and downs she had been a constant presence and had helped us keep order in our chaotic way of life.

Sean and Stacy had been a part of her life, as a sort of extended family, since they were in their early teens. She was a mother of sons and a daughter and felt our pain on a very personal level. It would be hard for her. I tried to make her comfortable and spend time with her until she could get used to what our future realities would be. I hoped she would hang in there with us.

How often Dolores and I had kidded about growing old together, sitting in rocking chairs on our great porch and telling stories about the good old days. We never thought the good old days would feel like this. Only good memories that would make us laugh were allowed. I couldn't control the cards that were dealt, but I felt blessed by having loyal, loving friends like Dolores. I hoped she knew how much I valued her friendship.

"Happy Birthday, Mom!" were the first words I heard on my forty-eighth birthday. Happy was not my feeling on that first day of September. The sweetness in Sean's selfless message was matched only by the bitterness of our present situation. Selflessness was becoming a new part of Sean's personality.

I tried desperately to act normally. We all seemed to need that right now. I couldn't do anything to scare him. He had to feel that there was hope and that he would get well. Stacy and Brock also took their cues from how I handled such things. Everyone was trying so hard to do and be whatever the others needed, almost like a game of who would blink first.

I kissed Sean goodbye for the day and headed to Rochester for a birthday lunch with Stacy and a few of my close friends. It took all the strength I could muster to be gracious and good-humored. I forced myself to go, thinking it would also be good for Stacy to be with other people and engage in normal conversation. It was nice to have a handful of good friends with good hearts. I was finding that not many people could deal with sickness. It seemed to touch them personally and made them back away.

It was almost unbearable to sit through idle conversation about trivial things and minor complaints. After only a short time I was ready to get home and check on Sean. It was a day of complex emotions, with everyone engaging in little conspiracies to surprise me, resulting in a strained festive atmosphere. But theirs were sweet intentions, and I played along despite a strong instinct to hide in a closest and never come out.

The sweetest of all was Sean—perhaps the only person celebrating my birthday with pure intentions. He was trying his hardest to participate, loving me, wishing me happiness, and not knowing that all I wished for on this birthday was his life.

I was finding that there was great comfort in the daily routines I had previously taken for granted. Our new routine of going to the hospital in Buffalo was not comforting. Sean's day included a stop at the oncology clinic, where the staff seemed cold and disconnected, then on to the chemo clinic where the nurses were warm and tried their best to make him feel like a real human being. The last stop was the pain clinic. The waiting room of the pain clinic would be filled with people in every stage of discomfort, all waiting for their turns to try to communicate their levels of pain in hopes that they would be given relief. I sat there feeling guilty that I was well and they were suffering. They were all my children at that moment, but I had nothing to offer them save for sympathy. It seemed so inadequate.

I looked at Sean's sickly, broken body and spirit and ached to cradle him in my arms. What was he thinking? I knew what I was feeling. In some gruesome fashion, I believe that if I could cause myself pain I wouldn't feel as guilty for being well while he was so terribly sick.

As we sat there I marveled at how stoic and patient they all were, waiting silently for their turn. Perhaps when you're so desperately ill and life hangs in the balance, resignation sets in and intellect and emotions are placed on hold.

"Sean Reynolds." I was up like a shot and helped Sean to negotiate the hallway to the examining room. Sean asked me what to expect, but I didn't know what was coming around the next bend, either. A doctor entered. She was a plain, no-nonsense woman, but at least she showed a little warmth. She had Sean's file in hand and seemed to have been thoroughly briefed on his case.

She asked Sean some questions about his pain levels. I had to resist the urge to answer for him. I kept forgetting he wasn't a little boy any longer. Sean explained to the doctor that, on a scale of one to ten with level one being the least pain and level ten the worst, he was at about seven.

She said that they would attempt to reduce his pain levels to one or two. She also explained that the best control drug is morphine.

Sean became agitated. He didn't want morphine. He was afraid of addiction. I must admit that it frightened me, too. The doctor smiled knowingly, as if she'd heard the same response a million times before. "I know that's what most people think, but we have learned that morphine is really a wonderful drug. It's natural, and therefore the body assimilates it quickly and easily. It also works in the most unique way. If a patient like Sean suffers from pain caused by cancer or other diseases, the body will only use what it needs for the pain. There is no addiction. If the body doesn't need as much and is doing better, the patient will not need as much morphine. If too much is present, often patients will experience side effects like bad dreams and will want to cut back on their own. Addictions result only when there is no real physical pain and a person is using the morphine just for a psychological escape."

She added, "I will prescribe morphine pills and we'll monitor the dosage based on Sean's needs. Don't be afraid to use them. The secret in pain control is to keep ahead of it. If you have pain, you're too late; you must take the pills on schedule."

Sean and I were relieved and fascinated to learn that morphine is a natural product and would work "naturally" on Sean's pain. Reliance on natural products such as herbs, vitamins, and homeopathic remedies has only recently received attention and acceptance from "traditional" medical practitioners.

The pain relief process that the doctor described proved to be true with Sean. When he had a mini-remission, he backed himself off the morphine.

Addiction is complicated. A person can be psychologically as well as physically addicted. If you are seriously ill, work with a qualified pain specialist for safe, effective pain relief.

FOUR

FALL AND FAITH

Another day, more phone calls. It was still so new to me. I could only make so many of them each day. It was too draining, too hard.

I rehearsed for every one of them. Each person had to be told in a way that helped him or her cope with the startling message. I had composed a list, in no particular order, of people in our lives who needed to know what was happening. On some days, I felt particularly brave and in control, and I could make several calls. On other days, I could only make one call, and I had to select very carefully from the list.

I struggled when I had to call Vicki, Sean's godmother. She and I had been friends since fourth grade. In the days when my dad was drinking and life at our house was upside down, Vicki's mother and father were like second parents to me. I would have done anything not to make that call. Vicki had experienced tragedies of her own. Her wonderful father had died many years before of leukemia, and Colin, her beloved brother, had only recently lost his own hard-fought battle with cancer at the age of forty-seven.

I picked up the phone to dial her number. My mind was racing ahead trying to figure out what I was going to say to her. I hadn't spoken to her in months. How could I just call her up and say, "By the way, Sean is dying."? Pensively listening to the rings, I hoped she wasn't there. On the third ring she picked up.

"Vicki?"

"Yes?"

"It's … "

She started to laugh, "Pam, it's you?"

I was taken aback. "Why are you laughing?"

"I was just thinking about you."

Vicki and I always had this sort of sixth sense about each other, even after all these years. As she prattled on, she became aware that I was strangely silent on the other end of the phone.

"OK, what's up? I can always tell when somthing is bothering you."

Without realizing it, I started to cry. "Vick, it's Sean. He's sick, really sick." The events of the past months poured out of me. I was shocked at the flood of emotion. I thought I had cried myself out weeks before. She asked questions, and I answered the best I could. We shared a few tears. Welling up with emotion, she said she had to hang up to gather herself together.

She would call me in a few days.

"Pam, tell my godson I love him."

I spoke with Steve Rodner, Sean's godfather. He and I had been friends for more than thirty years. He and his wife Judy had had their own run-ins with cancer. They recommended an organization called "Can Help," which accesses multiple databases and networks with doctors and cancer patients all over the world. Then they supply available information on specific cancers, the prognosis and any available medical and alternative treatments. I followed their good advice.

Can Help asked me to send medical information on Sean. They were familiar with Sean's cancer, and their prognosis was in general agreement with that of the other healthcare providers we had consulted.

The next day Brock and I drove Sean to the hospital for his chemo session. While Sean was having chemo, Brock and I scheduled a private meeting with his doctor. I asked about short-term expectations while Brock took notes. I was grateful that Brock had carried his trusted journalist's notebook along. Both of us are so predictable in our own way. Brock is methodical. I usually wing it.

The doctor seemed more relaxed, not so distant. As before, however, he offered not even a glimmer of hope for Sean's condition.

I asked about foods, herbs, and vitamins—quoting the American Cancer Society's recommendations. "Is there a diet or supplement you would suggest for Sean now that he has cancer?" I asked.

It seemed like a reasonable question. But he looked me straight in the eyes and said, "Those things can help prevent cancer, but don't waste your time now. It won't do any good." Nutrition and holistic medicines were apparently not part of his practice regimen.

The days went slowly by. I was so proud of Sean, fighting so gallantly for his life. His dignity and resolve impressed many. I sensed that his own opinion of himself had been elevated by his determined response to his disease.

I spoke to an herbalist recommended by the Can Help organization. A cancer survivor himself, he seemed very knowledgeable. There was something about him that made it easy to believe and trust him. He had a wealth of knowledge gained from the practices of an assortment of Indian medicine men, Chinese herbalists, and countless others who had discovered cancer-fighting properties in naturally occurring substances. He gave us names and phone numbers of people to contact. When I called the people he'd referred they provided me with helpful information and comfort. I found I was becoming receptive to new ideas, and opening my mind and imagination gave me a new sense of hope.

I explained that Sean had problems keeping food down and that the chemo corrupted his taste buds. Nothing tasted good to him. A herbalist suggested soaking his feet in a herbal solution twice a day. Soaking his feet sounded bizarre, but

when I asked why he said that many ancient cultures administered medications that way. Apparently the body can absorb
nutrients readily through the feet, so it was a good way to get
herbs into a patient, especially if they were having trouble
holding things down orally.

His knowledge about Sean's type of cancer impressed me.
We ordered the herbs.

As the days dragged on, the pressure of trying to help Sean
while keeping my eye on my businesses was taking its toll. I
realized I had to try to compartmentalize the demands of
my new life. Coming up the last weekend in September was
the annual AppleUmpkin Festival, and I had a big part in it.
One of western New York's largest festivals, it drew more than
20,000 people during its two days. Lit by gaslights, the town
of Wyoming gave all who visited the chance to experience
the gentleness of days gone by. Parades, pie-judging contests,
pancake breakfasts, and arts and crafts all shared the stage set
in our beautiful valley.

It was the busiest weekend of the year for our shops, café,
and the Cannonball Run Pub and was always a thrilling time.
The shoppers hummed traditional Christmas carols while enjoying the Christmas lights and displays. My staff was used to
me running through the building before we opened yelling
"Showtime everybody!" In the past I would be the first into
the village and the last to leave. My assumption was that if I
wasn't there making it happen, then nothing would.

This year the AppleUmpkin Festival was different for me.
I couldn't get out of bed. I wanted nothing to do with the
festival. I tried to motivate myself, but I could not convince
myself that it was worth all the effort. Huddling under the
sheets, ashamed of myself, I was hoping no one would notice
my absence. Later that day Brock came to check on me. Was I
all right? I explained I wasn't feeling well, not letting on that
I was too afraid to go. He understood, did not push, and left
me alone. For two days, I mostly stayed in bed, only getting

up to tend to Sean's needs. Sunday night came and, with twilight, I realized that the festival was over. Brock came into the bedroom to see how I was feeling. I asked him how our businesses did. To my amazement he said we had one of the best festivals ever. I was both thrilled and depressed. The world had kept on spinning without me. The shops and staff managed just fine. It was at that moment I realized that I was not as vital a component to things as I had once believed. It was liberating but, at the same time, depressing. Would I ever be able to get excited about anything again? Only time would tell. I was finding it awfully hard to concentrate on anything unrelated to Sean and our private drama.

Much of the time Sean was uncomfortable. Relief came in bursts of time—two hours here, three hours there—all morphine-induced. Chemo was constantly infused into his body from his CAD pump through a tube in his vein. He wore his little pump like a gunslinger wore his holster and pistol. I was fascinated by how we can become used to even the most abhorrent things. The blessed morphine was taken by mouth—one, two, or three—depending on pain levels and all closely monitored as if a time bomb were ready to explode at any moment. I was afraid to sleep, afraid Sean would wake up and need me.

We got into a grim routine—home nurses and chemo trips. There was a lot of time to think. Time was passing, and I had little recall of the everyday things that had once so occupied my waking hours.

One crisp autumn day the view from our front door was especially spectacular. The valley rolled out in front like ocean waves heading to the shore. The beautiful fall shades of red and orange were punctuated with golden corn stalks. Across the valley, on top of the hills, a great, dark cloud approached. A thunderstorm was heading our way. Sean would be thrilled. He loved thunderstorms and often complained about the lack of them in Los Angeles. I woke him just as a violent burst of thunder and a flash of lightning lit the sky. Before our eyes, in the distance, the clouds separated from the heavens as if God were smiling and pleased with his work. The golden beams of warm light shone like spotlights on the misty valley below. Suddenly our attention was drawn to the left side of the valley. An exquisitely defined rainbow was growing. We both gasped. A parallel rainbow developed behind it. It was magnificent. I'd never seen a double rainbow.

Two perfect rainbows, beautiful and intertwined—like Sean and me, linked together in that moment. We stood in awed silence together, sharing this spiritual moment.

The nights got colder as the days grew shorter. It was hard to get out of bed before the darkness lifted. There seemed to be a constant leaden haze over everything. Would the world ever be vivid and crisp and glistening again?

How could I run my businesses? How would I interact with friends and strangers? How could I be a good wife to Brock? A good mother to Stacy and Sean?

I was thinking thoughts I'd never thought before and opening new doors in my mind.

Now I began to ask the ultimate question: Why is the concept of a higher power and life after death so much a part of human consciousness?

I thought of conversations I had had with famed artist and costume designer Russell Patterson more than twenty years before. I could listen to him talk for hours about his rivalry with John Held over who really created the "Flapper Girl." He was a set designer for Florence Ziegfield and was at Fox Studios when Shirley Temple was discovered. Russell knew everyone in the glamorous old days of Hollywood and the silver screen. He was perhaps one of the dearest and most elegant men I had ever met—so bright, so creative, such a visionary.

Even though he was in his late seventies and very frail, he was magical and his mind was strong and open to everything. The wisdom of one of his many lessons was now so clear.

"Pammi, whatever the human mind can think is possible," he told me, and at last I understood.

As the days passed, we didn't see Stacy very much. She seemed preoccupied. My mother's instinct suspected there was more to it than the landfall of recent problems.

She was busy with her job and studies—maintaining a 4.0 grade point average at the graduate level. How did she stay focused? I began wondering if she was in denial. Was she shutting down emotionally? I asked her about it. Our talk provided insights of a very different kind. She told me that, one day, while in the local grocery store, she had heard two women talking in the next aisle. She didn't pay much attention until she heard one of them mention our name.

"Did you hear about the Yates's son?"

"No," another woman replied.

"Well, he has cancer. He's going to die."

"You're kidding."

"Why would I kid? It'll be good. Now they'll know what it's like to be like the rest of us."

As Stacy shared the story she began to sob. It was the first time she'd let me see her cry in a long time "Mom, what kind of people are they?" I tried to comfort her.

"Remember, Stacy, when your friends were astounded that we order out for pizza like they did? They thought we ate steak every night in the main dining room and dressed for dinner."

We laughed at how far from reality that was.

I hugged her and gently brushed her hair back on her forehead like I did when she was a baby. No explaining could make such a cruel act bearable. I watched her leave the room to go spend time with Sean and pretend nothing was wrong.

After being cooped up in the house for weeks, we received a welcomed phone call from old friends the McCurdys, Davises, and Nortons, who felt we needed a night out and asked us to

meet them at our favorite local restaurant, the Old Heidel-
berg. It offered the best German food this side of Germany.
We had settled into a routine of sorts at home, and Sean was
feeling well enough to visit with some of his friends, so we
agreed.

At first, I expressed reservations about going out, but
Brock insisted we keep linked to friends through this trying
time. Sean also encouraged us to do things. He said he felt
guilty that he had taken so much of our time and attention.
Sean was changing before our eyes. When he had been well,
he had always been so self-involved. Since his illness he had
become thoughtful and considerate. Now his first instinct was
to make sure the other person's needs took precedence over
his own. It was good to get out of the house that evening and
enjoy our friends' company and even have a few laughs. We
talked about current events and politics. Unfortunately, the
evening ended on a bit of a low note. The popular film at the
box office was *Philadelphia* with Tom Hanks, about a man dying from AIDS. Our friends were giving it rave reviews. Brock
and I sat quietly without comment. At one point, someone
asked me if I had seen it and, before even thinking, I quipped,
"I'm living it. Why would I want to see that?"

All went quiet. We all sat feeling uncomfortable, grappling
with my comment and its obvious truth. How could I have
faulted them for not understanding what was happening in
our lives, just a few miles down the road?

Sean's evening went more smoothly. His friends were
amazed at his courageous struggle with never an ounce of self-
pity. Beneath that costume of impending death was Sean's
gentle soul and sense of humor struggling harder and harder
to be appreciated. He wanted no pity, only to be loved.

The irony was that, before his illness, Sean measured everything by how it appeared on the surface. How hard it must
have been for him as his body changed—the disease having
its way. He was learning to work on relationships with family,
friends, and coworkers. Sean was amazed to find that people

admired his struggle, and he gained much-needed acceptance and understanding, based not on superficial criteria but on something much more significant. Something that could be called love.

My First Prayer

Now, all those "Now I lay me down to sleep, I pray the Lord my soul to keep," pleases and gimmes that had filled up my life to that point seemed almost laughable. I was about to have my first true dialogue with a power larger than anything I'd recognized before—a dialogue that bubbled up unbidden from the very depths of my being.

FIVE

MARKS

After his morphine was increased Sean slept deeply. He only came down from his room to soak his feet in the herbal solution and to get an occasional nibble. Food still didn't appeal to him.

Late one afternoon he shuffled into the kitchen looking to see if our secretary Barbara had gone. He was embarrassed to have others see him. By now he was so thin. He was always in pajamas with his Hickman pump at his side. The little hair he had left made him look prematurely old. Sean had been extremely depressed for a few days, so our verbal exchanges had been limited to "How are you feeling?" and "Can I get you anything?" He looked around and asked if Barb had gone. I told him she had just left a few minutes before. He said he wanted to do his herbal soak and didn't want anyone to watch him. We both headed into the laundry room where I helped to prepare the soak. It had become a time to socialize.

On this day, his comments rocked me. He said he was extremely depressed and said that if he was going to die he wished it would just be over with. I struggled to keep my composure. He had never mentioned death before. His depression, loneliness, and illness had obviously turned his personal need for answers and comfort inward, to the inevitable question, *Why me?*

"What do you live for, Mom?" he asked. "I bet you live because of the family and your love for us." After a brief hesitation he went on to say, "I wish I were spiritual. I wish I believed in God. The only time I prayed, I begged God to take away my pain. Instead, he gave me cancer."

I continued to fiddle mechanically with the herbal solution. Think … think. How do I respond? "Honey, you've been through so much and have so much going into your body. It must be depressing. Would you like to speak with someone about it?"

"Just what I need, Mom. More medications and another doctor."

He walked out and staggered back upstairs.

I began to feel panic and headed for my room. My bedroom had become my sanctuary, and I threw myself across the bed and, for the first time in a long time, erupted in tears.

Through my tears, my mind and heart began to search for something, someone, a higher power to reach out to.

Wanting to pray, I wondered who to pray to. I was a mother already mourning the approaching death of my child. But I was hardly a devoted Catholic, having left the church in my teens. Without being aware, I found myself talking to the Virgin Mary.

"Mary, is this my son's destiny? Maybe he wasn't meant to be here long? Maybe I shouldn't try so hard to keep him alive. I'll miss him so. It's not supposed to be like this. I'm supposed to die first. Please take me. Mary, if I only knew there was something more, I think I could let him go."

The following morning, Friday, November 12, I awoke with a start at around 8:45. Rushing to grab my clothing, I called to Stacy. We were scheduled to attend a business trade show in Rochester and had to be ready to leave in an hour. As I dressed I noticed carefully drawn markings on my right foot: swirls and spider-like patterns; fine lines and broad strokes; marks on the arch and on the inside of my right foot. The markings between my toes looked as if my toes had been carefully separated, one from the other, by whomever had made them. Pools of what appeared to be ink flooded the space between my toes. Instinctively I started to wipe it off with a washcloth. Suddenly, I stopped trying to wipe it away. It was something I needed to investigate further. Besides, if I wiped it all away, no one would believe me, including myself. It was precisely drawn, yet there was no ink on my hand, on my other foot, or on my pajamas.

I remember my mind darting around to get oriented. I felt repelled, awed, and confused all at the same time. I couldn't pull my thoughts together. I had never ever experienced a time in my life when I couldn't explain what was happening to me. It scared me and, yet, almost as if I were processing things on two levels, I instinctively knew it was alright and would become clear with time.

After a few moments I called out to Stacy and Brock to come and take a look. Ever the journalist, Brock grabbed his camera and took photos.

Because Stacy and I were going to be late for the trade show I finished dressing. The mystery would have to be solved later that evening when we returned home. That day I went through the motions of dealing with clients and customers but remained preoccupied with the mysterious markings.

I tried mightily to convince myself I had to have done it myself. Each time I came up with a scenario, it didn't make any sense. I innately knew I didn't have anything to do with it. But what or who did it, and why? It was strange to even think about something that had no easy explanation.

When we returned that evening I tried to remember all that had happened the night before. I showered at 11:30, read until 1:00, woke up at 4:30 and went into the front bedroom to read for an hour, then I fell asleep until the alarm went off.

If I had marked my foot, or if something else had, it would have had to have happened between 5:30 and 8:45 in the morning. Could I have been in an altered state of consciousness and done this to myself?

Sean spent Friday evening visiting with a friend and, when he arrived home, I was walking around without my socks and shoes. I did not want to risk rubbing the marking off. I told him about the events of the prior night, leaving out, of course, the part about talking to the Virgin Mary about his impending death. He, the ultimate agnostic, was puzzled but didn't dwell on it.

I followed Sean to his room. His few hours out had exhausted him, but I was grateful at that point that he could still drive and kept trying to live a normal life. He told me about his evening and how uncomfortable his friends seemed with him. It made him sad. Then he asked why the person who had drawn on my foot hadn't come to him if he was supposed to be the recipient of a message.

The only answer I could give was, "Sean, you are not always open-minded about matters of faith. You may not have been ready to accept it. Plus, you are on morphine; no one would believe you."

That evening Brock and I stayed up and talked about the drawings on my foot. He said that after I had headed off to the show he'd stripped all the linens off both beds and found no ink. He also pointed out that I'm right-handed. If I had done this to myself, I would have logically done it to my left foot, not my right. Images of my foot and this strange experience churned in my head. I kept trying to make some sense out of it. Everything told me I must have somehow done this to myself.

The next morning, after a long and sleepless night, I decided to drive to the Abbey of the Genesee—a well known Catholic monastery. It was a glorious, late fall day. A crisp chill smarted against my face as I started up the short pathway to the main entrance to the abbey. It was a rather severe building and did not look very welcoming. I didn't know what to expect, but I was drawn forward. The mystery of the markings seemed to call for a more spiritual answer.

I stood inside the abbey's main entrance. The dim light

and complete silence evoked in me a strange feeling. I wasn't
as comforted as I thought I would be. Off in the corner was
a small group of people who had come to purchase bread. It
was made at the abbey by the monks each morning and sold
to visitors as well as local markets.

I fidgeted around, hoping a monk would approach
me. When that didn't happen I decided to find someone. I
knocked on a closed door and a monk answered. He stood
about five-foot-nine and was dressed in casual clothes. He
asked me my reason for being there. He seemed standoffish
and unwelcoming. I was uncomfortable but decided to share
my story. I told him my son was dying of cancer and of my
unusual experience with my foot. He ushered me down a
long hallway and into a simple room devoid of anything but
a couple of chairs.

He looked uncomfortable, and I wondered if I had come
to the wrong place. When I removed my shoe and sock, the
monk pulled back. I managed to finish my story and looked
into his expressionless face for a response. After a few seconds
of thought he told me I should go to the police. I quickly put
on my shoe and sock and thanked him. He sensed my disap-
pointment and embarrassment. As I was leaving he called out
to me.

"I have a story to tell you. Quite a few years ago we had
a younger monk here. He had been ill with cancer for a long
time. We took turns caring for him and praying with him. As
death was approaching, he could no longer speak or respond
to us. I was with him at the moment of his death. He sat
bolt upright, opened his eyes, outstretched his arms toward
a picture of the Virgin Mary that hung at the foot of his bed.
He looked straight at her, smiled, and then died peacefully. I
witnessed it, so I know it happened. That's all I know."

I thanked him and silently took my leave.

As I walked down the abbey pathway toward my car, I noticed a statue of the Virgin Mary. I walked over to the grassy
spot where she stood vigil and got down on my knees, wept,
and prayed.

When I left the monk I was content with his story. Just accept what he said and leave things alone. I had an answer, maybe not exactly what I was looking for, but it should satisfy me. As I drove, however, the markings on my foot began to occupy my mind again. I had become a "doubting Thomas." My intellect was still demanding a real-world explanation. I needed to know if there was one.

I felt I had to show my foot to someone I could trust, someone outside our family circle who could witness that it really happened and wasn't a figment of my imagination.

Bob and Arianna Davis popped into my mind. We had been friends for many years. Bob was a pragmatic business-man and Arianna an academic. Arianna had an interest in the paranormal and mystical while Bob was more practical. They might be a perfect choice to help solve my mystery.

As I pulled into the driveway to their three-story Victori-an home, I had no way of knowing that this would be another of many roads that I would travel in my search for answers. Their good-natured black Lab welcomed me and ushered me up the steps leading to the back door near their kitchen.

The smell of a fresh baked apple pie welcomed me as I entered their kitchen. Arianna is a great cook and spoils her family and friends with her marvelous desserts and traditional, old-world recipes. She was always comforting to be around. Positive, upbeat and extremely resourceful, Arianna has always been someone I admire. Bob, with his dry sense of humor, was very grounded and could be counted on for his honesty.

I explained the reason for my visit. "You are the only friends I have shared this with." As we all moved to take our seats at the kitchen table, I began to explain the events of the past few days. I told them about my conversation with Sean about death and my desperate prayer to the Virgin Mary. When I finished I showed them my foot and the markings. The room was silent. Then they both responded. Each had their own thoughts about what they were witnessing.

Arianna was intrigued and excited. Bob admitted that, before he even saw the markings he was sure I must have made them; but once he saw them he was no longer convinced. We went over the details of my story at length. I left their home, however, with more questions than answers.

Needing to get back to work, I headed to the Christmas Shoppe and spent the rest of the day with customers. I finally arrived home, exhausted and still struggling to come to terms with what had happened to me.

By the third morning I was getting used to the mysterious markings on my foot. Brock remained as intrigued as I. The monk's comments kept going through my mind—"Go to the police." I resisted doing that but kept wondering if the strange pen Brock had found on his desk the morning we discovered the markings had been used to make them. The color of the ink matched; it was a felt tip calligraphy pen and that certainly seemed to explain how the lines were wider in some places and thinner in others. Neither of us recognized the pen as one we owned nor had any idea how it came to rest on Brock's desk.

Sean was also caught up in the mystery. He kept asking me to remove my sock and show him the markings. We mused together about the possibility that it could be a paranormal experience. After a while, we joked about the what-ifs. At one point he said, "I always thought you were out of this world, but really Mom!"

By Sunday night Brock noticed how distracted I was becoming. He suggested I call an acquaintance of his who was a lieutenant with the police.

I was still self-conscious and a bit embarrassed, but the next day I called the lieutenant and set up an appointment. I thought I'd bring him the washcloth with the ink and the suspect pen to see if they could run tests to determine if the pen caused the markings. On Tuesday we met. After showing him my foot I gave him the evidence. He, too, was astounded, but he said it was against department regulations to use the lab for personal reasons. If I promised not to tell anyone, he said he would have someone in the forensic lab check it out and he would get back to me if they found something. He took another look at my foot and left.

By Thursday I'd been struggling for almost a week with how and why the markings had appeared on my foot I wasn't about to wash my foot and have them disappear without the chance to try and find out what had happened. All the obvious possibilities had been exhausted. I believed that the only thing left was for me to be hypnotized. I called my friend who was a prominent psychiatrist. He told me about another psychiatrist from a university nearby who was an experienced hypnotist.

I called to schedule an appointment, and when his nurse asked my reason for seeing the doctor I told her my story, with much embarrassment. She expressed some shock and amusement but seemed interested in having me meet with the doctor. She told me not to remove the markings from my foot and to come in to the office on Monday. He was busy but, because of the unusual circumstances, would make time for me that day.

During the weekend as I waited for my appointment, Brock, Sean, and Stacy became impatient with me because I kept trying to set up scenarios to explain the markings. I was trying everyone's patience. We all wanted the mystery to end.

I did receive some reassurance during those days from our friend at the police department. He called and asked if I would come back and meet with him and the head of the forensic lab, a recent transplant from the NYPD. This burly, seasoned police investigator had seen a lot, but this case seemed to puzzle him. He returned the pen and washcloth, telling us the tests confirmed that the ink on my foot had indeed come from the pen, but no fingerprints were found. Nor was there any other evidence to point to how the markings had been made or by whom. It remained a mystery, even to the police.

When I arrived at the doctor's office his nurse asked me to expose my foot. I felt embarrassed taking off my sock in front of a total stranger. She gasped when she saw how well defined the markings were. Then she led me into one of the examination rooms. When the doctor entered he seemed mild-mannered and extremely professional.

He wasted no time in small talk. He looked at my foot and expressed surprise at the detail and neatness of the markings, saying he'd never seen anything quite like it before. He asked me some perfunctory questions about myself and Sean. I explained in detail the events of the night the markings appeared on my foot. He sat silent, never revealing any emotion.

He asked, "Have you ever before experienced a fugue state?"

"Fugue state? What's that?"

"When you lose time and your mind takes a holiday from your body." I was taken aback with the reality of what he was implying.

"No, never. Not to say I haven't thought of that myself, but I have never walked in my sleep or even talked in my sleep. As a matter of fact, I am a very light sleeper."

"I don't believe in the paranormal," he said firmly. "As a scientist I cannot."

He was getting more conversational and I was fascinated by his information.

"I'm not sure I do, either. I am perfectly willing to discover that I did this to myself. Frankly it would be a great relief. The only thing I do know is that I don't feel connected to this event."

"Well," he said, "Let's get started. Have you ever been hypnotized?"

"A couple of times in the past. I've been told I'm a good subject," I replied.

He got out of his chair, closed the blinds, turned on his tape recorder. He used the pendulum method to put me under. I had forgotten how strange a sensation it was. It felt totally normal, as if I were in control, even to the point of questioning whether I was really hypnotized. All of a sudden, the doctor was questioning me and tears were streaming down my checks and words and emotions were pouring out. The doctor took me through some routine questions about my life and our present situation with Sean. It felt good to release some of that pent-up emotion. He walked through the day, in case I had forgotten anything. To my surprise the story was so clear to me I knew I hadn't buried anything.

"Tell me about bedtime. What were you thinking and what did you do?" he asked.

I remember pausing to think, but then the words just flowed out of my mouth.

"I took a shower and put on my pajamas. I didn't see any markings then. I got into bed at 11:30. I fell asleep. Awoke about 4:30 in the morning. Then I went into the small front bedroom and read until around 5:30. Still, nothing unusual. I fell asleep and awoke at 8:45. I raced into the bathroom to get dressed, glanced down, and gasped at the marks on my foot."

Back and forth we went. He kept quizzing me about those hours. He came at me from every possible direction but each time he went to the foot, my mind went blank. I couldn't tell him a thing. He seemed frustrated with me because he was convinced that I had done it to myself. As a last resort, he put a pad in my hands with a pencil and took me through the events again and again, hoping my hand would try to recreate the markings. Nothing, absolutely nothing. No luck. With that he brought me out of hypnosis. Finally he said to me, "How long do you think you've been under?"

I thought and replied, "About twenty minutes."

He replied firmly. "It's been an hour and a half."

I was startled at the amount of time I'd been there.

After a moment's reflection the doctor said, "I don't know what to tell you, but I strongly believe you did not do this to yourself." He said that, if by some chance I had, as time went on and things with Sean got worse, I would act out again. It wouldn't be a one-time thing. He said "When you go to bed tonight, you should try and recreate that evening."

I said, "I'll try."

He ended his interview with, "Do you know anyone who deals with the paranormal?"

I was surprised at this statement and I told him that I did not. "I thought you said you didn't believe the paranormal."

"As a scientist I don't believe," he paused "But there is a scientific category we call 'not proven'." He said he believed that my situation fell into that category and reiterated that he'd never seen anything quite like it. He wished me well and told me to keep in touch and let him know if anything else happened.

I promised I would try and left even more confused than before. Tears broke as I walked to my car; the tension and confusion finally sunk in. What was I to think? It was my last hope for putting this behind me and now it would haunt me forever.

It was important to try to put it behind me, however, at least for awhile. Thanksgiving was only three days away and it might be our last with Sean. I started to prepare the feast. Exhausted and fractured, I did the best I could, considering the circumstances. I wasn't sure what would taste good to Sean due to the medications he was taking. He was eating so little. As I prepared, I exhorted myself to make it memorable, keep it upbeat, be a good wife and a good mother to Stacy and Sean.

It was important that life seem normal for Sean even though it was anything but. I kept remembering what someone had told me, that God gives you only what you can handle.

I had my doubts.

Thanksgiving arrived and I shuffled down at the crack of dawn to put the stuffing in the turkey. Knowing I wasn't a morning person, Sean and Stacy would kiddingly remind me to make sure the turkey's less desirable parts were removed before I stuffed it. My concern was making sure that I had calculated the time correctly so that we could eat on time.

Thanksgiving has always been my favorite holiday, a chance to be with family and friends around a table loaded with decadent yet delightful foods. The shared conversations around the dinner table remained part of the magic and tradition of the holidays.

Ever since we had opened the Gaslight Christmas & Holiday Shoppe it had become a much loved destination for many Christmas shoppers. On Thanksgiving weekend, the village and our shops filled to overflowing with people hoping to capture the sweetness of days gone by. It was the start of a month of excitement and anticipation, of traditions, foods, music, and the little secrets building up to Christmas. For me, as for many, November and December are the most romantic months of the year.

This was the first holiday since Sean's diagnosis. It had a dynamic all its own. It was a reality check. This could be Sean's last Thanksgiving. I couldn't imagine such a thing.

That Thanksgiving morning I was motivated to make it a wonderful and memorable dinner. I went over my menu endlessly to make sure I didn't forget a thing.

One of our family traditions was that each person could request one of their favorite foods. Everybody agreed on the basics—turkey, mashed potatoes, gravy—but the rest of the meal was by request. Brock asked for acorn squash, my mother apple pie, my father candied sweet potatoes, Stacy corn soufflé and last, but not least, Sean wanted Mom's famous popovers. He loved watching them pop and get gloriously brown in the oven. I must admit it was always fun for me to serve them and have everyone relish and enjoy them.

That Thanksgiving day was truly a day of blessings for us. Sean awoke feeling pretty good and vibrating with excitement about the holiday. He wandered into the kitchen around eleven, sniffing the wonderful cooking smells. He gave me a great big hug. "Wow, Mom, it smells great!" I put my arms around him, resisting the urge to cry, and said, "I hope you like it, or you might replace me." Sweetly, he whispered, "You? Never, Mom." Luckily, my parents arrived just then. I don't think I could have kept from weeping if we had remained alone.

My parents were in great spirits. My father, the kidder, began his usual ragging on Sean: "Hey Seanie give your old grandfather a kiss." This elicited an embarrassed response from Sean, but he loved my dad and played along.

"Oh, Papa. I'm going to be forty and you're still going to call me Seanie?"

Dad's retort: "Hey, getting too big in your boots to give the old boy a kiss?"

My mother, on the other hand, was the no-nonsense, let's-get-the-show-on-the-road sort. She busied herself with pre-paring food and keeping the kitchen in ship shape. Brock tried his best to stay out of the way during the fixing of the meal, but after dinner he could always be counted on to say, "You girls made a great dinner; now the guys will do the dishes." It was truly a family affair.

This Thanksgiving day seemed to have an extra helping of positive energy. It was as if Sean, and all the rest of us, had rallied because we knew that it was a must-be-special, *precious* time for all of us. Even the turkey cooperated and made its appearance at the correct time. It was a wonderful meal. Sean even managed to get more food down than he had in weeks. At the end of the day, the mood was far different from what I had anticipated. Everyone had either gone home or to bed and I was relishing the quiet time alone as I put away the sil-ver service and dishes.

It had been a lovely day, poignant and bittersweet as most profound experiences are. The table looked wonderful and, among our small group of immediate family, the love could be felt. We usually had many friends over, but I knew that with everyone but Sean knowing how serious his illness was I couldn't impose that burden on them and place a pall on their holidays. It was okay, though. It was fitting. There were even some humorous moments when the food kept coming out and the variety of dishes exceeded that of a White House banquet. I never really considered the numbers to be served, only that I had to make every dish each family member had ever expressed a liking for. It was overkill to say the least, but we managed to make a big dent in it anyway.

As I wandered the dining room, I was proud of my family. They carried the day with grace and courage. I was sure they all struggled in their own ways. I also know on this day of Thanksgiving they each must have overcome sadness to find reasons to be thankful. I know I did.

SIX

CHRISTMAS

When Thanksgiving was over, the days grew shorter, but my chats with Sean became longer. We continued to grow closer. I learned more about his childhood and his confusion and anger with his biological father as he opened doors to his past. I was always puzzled as to why he and Stacy never wanted to visit their father. He would often drop out of their lives for months, even years, at a time. Neither Sean nor Stacy revealed much about the time they spent with him. I always believed it was their loyalty to him that kept that part of their life experience from me. I learned that it was out of concern for me that they didn't share these experiences.

Because of his illness, Sean had endless hours to rethink his life. He was trying to come to terms with his own feelings about his father. He revealed that, in his early teens, he hated to visit his father because he would take Stacy and Sean to his favorite bars. They were uncomfortable because they saw and heard things they were ashamed of. I was horrified but tried not to show much emotion. I expressed my shock and regrets for them both, but it was terribly hard to walk that fine line between sympathetic confessor and indignant, protective mother. Sean seemed to be relieved to be able to share his anger, finally. Certainly he was more at peace with himself and learning to be more reflective. He had decided to "use his time wisely." One of his new missions was to learn to use a computer. His company had promised to keep his job open until he could return. He had spoken with his friend and co-worker Dennis and was making plans to work at home. Brock and I were so grateful to them for their kindness. They knew as we did that Sean would never return to work, but like us they wanted to keep Sean's hope alive.

To my astonishment, Sean decided to go to Rochester alone and was very secretive about his trip. When he returned, he announced he had been to a doctor whose name I had found for him, a highly respected psychiatrist. Sean was fighting hard to survive.

"Well," I said, "How did it go? How did you like him?"

"It was okay. I liked him. I plan to go every week until I get better."

I was so thankful! He needed to let his feelings out.

Just prior to Christmas I met a psychologist friend for lunch. She was interested in seeing the photos of the markings on my foot. I told her the story of my day with Sean and my prayer to the Virgin Mary. Pulling out the pictures she looked for a moment and then said, "The color of the ink!"

I asked, "What about it?"

She said, "That color blue is the color associated with the Virgin Mary."

That was something I had never thought about. Even though she no longer participated she had been a Catholic.

I asked if she believed in the paranormal.

She said quietly, "Yes I do."

The discussion that followed was stimulating. It was wonderful exploring the possibilities—of angels, life after death, out-of-body experiences, all the mysteries of life that people silently struggle with. It was liberating for me to be able to share and discuss my thoughts.

One day Sean drove to Rochester. He had been using our SUV because it had an automatic transmission and was easier for him to drive than his car, which had a stick shift. When he returned home, the SUV was loaded with boxes. I was astonished. As frail as he was, he carried the large boxes into the house. He was so excited. On his trip he had purchased a new television, video recorder, and an entertainment center. Sean was never known for his patience in building things. Usually he got frustrated and couldn't wait to have someone else finish. I felt the urge to discourage him from attempting to put those heavy pieces of wood together because he was so frail. Brock thought it was more important to him to feel normal and enthusiastic than to protect him and make him feel he was too ill.

It was a great day! Sean assembled his entertainment center, and he was elated. His hard work had paid off. To our amazement, he loved every minute of it and never once got frustrated. I continued to marvel that out of great tragedy and sorrow came many positive surprises. Sean decided that when he was better he would take some classes in woodworking. We were witnessing a metamorphosis.

It was ten days before Christmas, and the pressures of work, shopping, dealing with Sean's illness and our own fears about the future were taking hold. Would this be our last Christmas together? It was an impossible concept to get our minds and hearts around. Here was this young man—twenty-six years old, our son, Stacy's brother—who would not be here next year.

We had always looked forward to the Christmas holidays with such joy, and now we were dreading that they would come too quickly. Sean's main concern was finding the perfect gift for everyone, especially Stacy. He said he felt guilty that he was buying all these great things for himself and Stacy didn't even have a good stereo. We were all bound up by what we knew, and Sean was living his own reality. He had become so gentle and considerate, so interested in the happiness of others. Was it a result of his counseling, or had he experienced a transformation? Whatever it was, he was changing dramatically with each passing day. I guess we don't choose when and how we learn our lessons.

I was also pleased for Stacy. She desperately needed to know that Sean loved her, and finally he was showing it.

A week before Christmas I had lunch with a doctor from Rochester. I had arranged to meet him about a fundraiser that I had committed to long before Sean became ill. I didn't want to back out of another commitment and go through the painful retelling of our family's tragedy. Did I dare show him the pictures of the markings on my foot?

It took about a half-hour to muster the courage. After I showed him the photos I asked his opinion. He studied the pictures and then paused. To my astonishment, he said that his mother had great psychic abilities. Being raised with the sense that paranormal experiences were real was what led him to explore science and medicine. He said that there are many things we cannot see with the naked eye, such as the atom, electricity, and sound, but they certainly exist. "Pam, we are only limited by our own ability to see and understand. I believe your markings and story have all the makings of a paranormal experience. Don't be ashamed to let yourself believe what I think you seem to know in your heart. I have known you a long time as a patient and as a person. If you truly feel something or someone reached out to you from another dimension, trust your instincts."

Christmas was almost upon us and, for the first time in my life, I truly grasped the profound importance of traditions. In the past our favorite family tradition was the annual tree-trimming party. Family and close friends gathered to decorate the tree, share eggnog and cookies, and sing Christmas carols. This year was different. Rather than a large party we kept it to just our family. Sean, Stacy, Brock, my mother, and I decorated the tree. We laughed at the tacky old ornaments and silly memories of Christmases past. It was a magical night.

Earlier we had brought the tree home, which was a comedy in itself. We must have looked funny when our car manuevered its way up our street, buried under the weight of a giant fir tree. There was only one problem: We couldn't lift it off the roof of the car. After enlisting several friends we finally were able to carry the tree into the house.

As several helpers placed the tree into its stand, I helped to make sure it was tall and straight. It looked like the raising of the tree at Rockefeller Center. The Fraser fir's branches were coarse, cutting our skin with each touch. As I was lying on my back under the tree trying to hold on while it was moved into position, I began to itch all over. I couldn't see it at that moment but I had broken out in hives and couldn't scratch the itching. I was allergic to the tree.

Suddenly the giant tree lunged forward, snapping the twine binding it to the staircase railing. The huge width of the lower branches had spread out, filling the center hall to overflowing. There was almost no room for the furniture, let alone the gifts. The sheer weight of the Fraser fir had crushed the tree stand, releasing the water all over the center hall floor. Needless to say, our Christmas spirit took a short holiday and everyone wanted to kill *me* because I had been the one to demand the largest tree possible. Now the tree had to be secured to prevent it from crashing into the chandelier and taking the staircase with it. As usual, Sean's wonderful ability to see the absurdity of situations saved the day. He began regaling us with the classic funny vignettes from our favorite silly movie "The Money Pit." Once the tree was secure we all spread out on the center hall floor, laughing and making fun of my "superb" choice of trees.

The tree was so majestic in the otherwise darkened center hall.

I must admit, it was the largest, most beautiful tree we ever had—fourteen feet high and almost as wide. Brock and I must have walked three miles to find it. It was set in a clearing in the farthest corner of the tree farm, all alone, regal and proud. It broke my heart to cut it down, but this Christmas was to be special; we needed its beauty and splendor. It would be the last Christmas tree Sean would ever see.

We wanted to make Christmas last a lifetime for the entire family. The food, the music, the tree, the love—all must last in our memories. Everyone was fussing about, wrapping their secret treasures, focusing on someone else's happiness. It was a great feeling. But despite the holiday cheer, I felt especially sad for my mom. She had spent a good part of her life tending to her sisters, brother, and cousins while each fought the cancer that would take their lives. Cancer seemed to plague her mother's side of the family. Realizing the next person to be taken from her was her grandson was almost more than she could bear. As I watched her spend time with Sean, and help with his care, I never loved her more.

For several weeks Sean had been feeling much better. He seemed so content to wrap his presents and be in the safety of our home.

I hadn't been to church in years. This year I felt the need to go to midnight mass and take heart from the joy and inspirational atmosphere that permeated the inside of the church.

Then it was Christmas morning, my favorite day of the year. I was so grateful we had been given the time to spend it all together and that, by some miracle, Sean was feeling well enough to be joyful.

First, I made the coffee and put out the muffins while my Mother placed the chairs around the tree that had miraculously exploded with gifts while we were all asleep. I secretly put the last little gifts in Sean's and Stacy's Christmas stockings and figured that, by ten o'clock, I could wake them without enduring much grumbling. Surprisingly, Sean was moving around on his own and Stacy, too, was ready to come down and greet the day.

Music on, cameras out, our little family gathered, each heart dealing in its own way with that final Christmas. Sean was so excited about his gifts to Stacy that all else paled. I don't think he realized just how much the love and caring transcended the gifts. It wasn't just a gift for Stacy, but to all of us. When I think of it, it is perhaps the best and truest Christmas we'd ever shared.

SEVEN

WINTER OF OUR DISCONTENT

While Christmas was filled with so much joy, New Year's Day was the opposite. No one wished us a Happy New Year. No one could, knowing what the new year would bring to us. I puzzled about what my resolution would have been if I had felt inclined to make one. Maybe there were too many to count. Perhaps I couldn't settle on one because I was too afraid of failing. Where would we all be next New Year? How would Sean's passing change our lives and each of us? It was too much for me to contemplate.

Brock and I went to our condo for a few days just to get away. It was so good to be in a different environment—another game of pretend.

I found myself dialing a psychic hot line. It was crazy. I was curious to see how much they could guess right. While trying not to reveal anything that they could use to impress me, I was still trying to find out anything I could about my foot. It had become a search for my personal Holy Grail.

Her name was Mira and she seemed appropriately exotic while very pleasant and easy to talk to. She asked pretty standard questions about me. We talked of general things. She never even got close to Sean's illness, let alone my foot markings. Good try, I thought—myself and ten million others looking for answers. At the end of the conversation I revealed that our son was dying of cancer and she instantly departed from her scripted routine and gave me a number to call. She spoke softly. "Call this man who lives in Arizona," she said. "He is an Indian medicine man who has achieved some good results with an exotic tea mixture." I took the number gratefully because, when terminal cancer is a part of your life or that of someone you love, you are open to try anything.

Sean began to complain of back pain again. I feared his little remission was coming to an end. The telltale signs were there: his inability to stand for very long, loss of appetite, and bowel problems. The realities and the fear of the future returned with a vengeance.

On top of this, Sean had decided to visit a friend in Boston. He was so intent on making the trip, no one had the heart to talk him out of it. It was important that he continue to feel he had a future. While the travel would be hard on him, it was important for him to go. Besides, it was the first effort he had made to do something enjoyable since Christmas.

By February I couldn't sleep, although Sean seemed fairly comfortable. My days and nights were all mixed up. I couldn't sleep even when I got the chance because I was afraid he would need me.

One night, just past midnight, I turned on the television to an episode of *Unsolved Mysteries*. It was a segment dealing with the paranormal, a very credible episode. I tried calling the show to talk to one of their experts. Perhaps, I hoped, I could arrange for a paranormal expert to visit our home. I might learn more about the markings on my foot. It showed how desperate one can become when looking for answers to something unexplained.

A few weeks later, Sean's condition started to change. I knew the cancer was now spreading rapidly. He was sleeping more and had increased his morphine dose. Time itself lost its meaning. Life was now on "Sean time." I was becoming task-oriented—needing specific tasks to focus on to keep my sanity. I became a cleaning machine—tackling one room in the house at a time, cleaning everything from top to bottom. Soon I was running out of rooms to tackle. We were a fort in hostile territory. It was us against the disease. We went nowhere because we wouldn't leave Sean. I cleaned because it was the only thing I seemed to be able to control.

February 4 was Stacy's birthday. Her college graduation the previous May seemed like ancient history. I daydreamed about what path she would have taken had she not gotten sidetracked by her brother's illness. Brock and I, as we did with all the children, talked of her future and her dreams. I was so sorry we couldn't share a happy evening exchanging gifts and old stories, but it would have been too forced—too tough. Her courage and dignity took my breath away. Never had I been prouder of the woman she'd become.

I felt I had to get away, to take a break from the oppressive weight of Sean's struggle. As with most things, this seemed to be an easy, sensible remedy that was much more complex in the doing. My mind wrestled with the concept that he was doing the suffering and I was the one needing to get away for some peace.

But it was also obvious that the stress and tension were taking a toll on Brock's and my relationship. We were trying to be strong for each other without showing our own personal emotions and fears. It was an unnatural situation compounded by having to put a happy face on for Sean's and Stacy's benefit. With the blessing of both Sean and Stacy, Brock and I went to our home in the Thousand Islands for a brief getaway.

We had been vacationing there for years. When we had our sportfishing boat, we would cruise from Shumway's Marina, in Rochester, to Alexandria Bay and spend two weeks on the St. Lawrence River. We had grown to love the area so much that in 1991 we purchased a three-story condominium overlooking Boldt Castle. Boldt Castle was designed and created in 1893 by George Boldt, founder of the famous Waldorf

Astoria Hotel, in New York City, for his beloved wife. Inspired by the extraordinary architectural buildings created for
the world renowned Chicago World's Fair of the same year,
Boldt chose to recreate a magnificent castle like the ones on
the Rhine River he remembered from his youth in Germany.
To this day, it remains a wondrous surprise as it rises majesti-
cally out of the St. Lawrence River.

As it always was for Brock and me, the sight of the Thousand Islands Bridge was so welcoming as it arced its way
across the St. Lawrence wearing its glittering lights like a thin
diamond bracelet between the United States and Canada.
Beneath is the majestic river hosting freighters from exotic
ports-of-call such as Singapore, Liverpool, and Hong Kong.
The commerce of the world floats up and down the river
with flags flying a silent salute to all like me who watch and
dream of adventure and mysterious surprises. How that part
of me that was not Sean's mother longed to stow away and
flee—never to look back, never to deal with the cruel realities
that awaited me.

Brock and I were always at peace in the Thousand Islands.
It's a place of endless beauty, and that beauty nurtured us. I
supposed part of my personal journey was to learn to accept,
to balance life's forces, and to make myself ready to help Sean
and my family cope with our impending loss. If I'm all right,
they will ultimately be all right, too, I reasoned.

The nights were even harder in the Thousand Islands than
at home. I walked the floors, couldn't sleep. My heart was
with Sean. Sometimes it was harder to take comfort in the
tranquility than to be in the trenches fighting the war. The
night sky there was vast. The heavens showcased the millions
of stars and planets. As the sky met the St. Lawrence River,
the ceaseless current, with its incalculable power, held me in
thrall. There is a great plan, a greater power, it whispered.

Weren't a few years of having Sean to love—and then
lose—better than having never known him? I was realizing
that the quality of a life well lived far transcends its length.

A light snow was falling as I looked across the water at Boldt Castle through the mist. It was always a magical experience for me. It took me back to the old *Wonderful World of Disney* television show when Jiminy Cricket would open with the song "When You Wish Upon a Star." In those days, my wishes were a lot smaller and simpler. I do remember thinking that they were every bit as unattainable.

Brock came up from behind, startling me as he put his arms around my waist, "Can I ask the most beautiful girl in the world for a date?"

Feeling the love and warmth of his arms around me, I replied, "I would love to spend an evening with the man I love."

It felt so refreshing to get dressed in a lovely dress and high heels, put my makeup on my rather tired looking face. Moments like these were the only times I was grateful that the aging process brought with it diminished visual capacity. In Brock's eyes, I still looked good after all these years.

Brock had arranged for a lovely candle-lit dinner at a little restaurant called Chez Piggy in Kingston, Ontario. Just across the Thousand Islands Bridge on the Canadian side, it was started by one of the owners of the Lovin' Spoonful singing group. We had a great dinner and talked as if we hadn't seen each other in years. We realized that we had been so mired in the talk of illness that we were losing the art of normal conversation. We were craving normalcy and laughter. We both agreed we had to try to make time for each other even if it was only for a few hours each week.

When we arrived back at the condo I closed the door to lock it, and Brock took me in his arms and kissed me. It was so wonderful to feel desirable and alive. I changed into my prettiest nightgown and splashed on his favorite perfume. I took a fast look into the mirror, and was surprised at how tired I looked. I climbed into bed and snuggled up to Brock. His arms enveloped me. I was lost in the moment. But, as he tenderly kissed me, I pulled away abruptly and began to cry.

"Why are you crying? What's the matter?"

"I just realized Sean is home alone and we are up here having a lovely time. I can't make sense of it. It's like I have this mental checklist: Sean, Stacy, you, shopping, laundry, and my businesses. Brock, my son is dying and I must do my best to care for him." Romance seemed to be out of the question just then.

Upon our return home we started to have dinner together each night. "Together" those days meant Brock, Stacy, and me. Sean slept. He couldn't eat, so I didn't cook. I use the word *dinner* loosely because I had stopped cooking months before. I didn't want the food smells to reach him and make him unhappy.

Gone were the enjoyable creative menus I so loved to conjure up. Unlike many, I loved to grocery shop and hurry home to whip up some exotic recipe. Brock, who is such a good sport, would have to pretend he loved it. Although he was easy to please, I often tested his good temper and adventuresome taste buds. I became the most creative salad-maker on the planet. I figured salads don't give off odors. Pizza was the only delivery option in our rural location. Up until that point in our lives, we thought we could never get tired of pizza. But, like the old saying goes, "Be careful what you wish for—you may get it."

We had begun to live in parallel universes. Our abbreviated little family of Stacy, Brock, and me tried to create a "normal" day-to-day existence. We would eat dinner, such as it was, and talk about current events, business happenings, and sometimes local gossip. Our other life with Sean was filled with medical information, procedures, pretense, and sometimes, if Sean was feeling a bit better, precious exchanges of love and life. I now realized how we had all taken the family moments of simple pleasures and exchanges for granted.

February 18. Our wedding anniversary! Seven months into this nightmare, and Brock and I almost forgot our own anniversary. We wouldn't even have remembered if we hadn't found Stacy's sweet card. My parents sent a card, too. Poor Mom and Dad! They didn't know what to do. It was inconceivable to them that Sean was dying. The natural order of life and death became scrambled. There was no logic to it.

As the day progressed and the monotony of our grim routine was grinding away at my stamina and patience, I began to realize I was getting angrier and angrier. Like an animal caught in a trap, I wanted to lash out at somebody—anybody.

I began stewing over the orthopedist in California, wanting to make him pay for Sean's pain. I called a lawyer who handled malpractice claims and learned that, in the legal profession, at least, there was even a formula for the value of life. I couldn't believe what I learned:

If the plaintiff in a lawsuit is a wife, child, or children of the deceased or injured, they refer to actuarial charts to determine how old the victim is or was and compare the age to the expected lifespan and also how much they could have possibly earned during that time.

If the victim is a baby or child the value of life is much less because they are considered non-producers or contributors.

If the victim is terminally ill the legal system says "too bad."

After speaking with lawyers in New York and Los Angeles about the legitimacy of a lawsuit against Sean's doctor in L.A. they gave me the following advice:

If your son is terminally ill and he was misdiagnosed, the courts and the insurance company will chew you up and spit you out because he is dead already. If *you* are misdiagnosed and it affects your quality of life and you're lucky enough to survive, the legal system is prepared to compensate you.

The logic posed some questions for me:

Doesn't the pain and suffering of the terminally ill have value? Doesn't the emotional anguish and inability to fulfill last dreams and wishes due to malpractice for the terminal patients have as much meaning as they do to someone who has the gift of life? Doesn't the realization that a doctor put you through unnecessary surgery and suffering and robbed you of precious time count for something? Isn't the quality of one's death, which we all face, not as important as the quality of that person's life? If the quality of one's death has so little value, especially if the patient is terminally ill, why are we as a society so opposed to doctor-assisted suicide?

These are all questions the system seems to either refuse to acknowledge or to which it simply quotes the formula of one's earning potential. How absurdly black and white and so inhumane!

Now one day became much like the next. Unless the news featured a new medical event, the global problems and local gossip held no interest and had no bearing on our lives. Sean and I would spend his awake time talking about anything and everything that happened to pop into our minds, almost in stream-of-consciousness conversations. He had always enjoyed his time with our family dogs and, being an animal lover, he watched endless Discovery Channel programs.

As I came into the room, he announced that a new English Mastiff puppy might be just the thing he needed to help his recovery. I stopped in my tracks and laughed out loud. "Sean, could you possibly have picked a larger dog?" We had owned a Mastiff named Rudy for years. He was named after the famous race driver Rudy Carociola—Brock's idea, of course. Rudy was the love of our family. He was 200 pounds, kind, smart, loyal, and very protective of Sean and Stacy. I didn't need another responsibility and certainly not one that size. "Oh. Mom, come on. You know you'd love one." All I could think of was Sean thinking it would help him recover. How could I say no?

Soon we had a new addition to our family, a Mastiff puppy the size of most full-grown dogs. Thirty of the cutest pounds I'd ever seen.

The dog was purchased sight unseen from a breeder and shipped by air to us. Poor Brock didn't even know he was going to be a proud new father. The Rochester baggage claim might never be the same after our sweet little puppy arrived, drawing a crowd of dozens.

Sean desperately wanted that Mastiff puppy. If he had wanted an elephant, I'd have found one. He could barely stay up for more than a few minutes at a time now, but he was so excited; each moment of joy was worth everything.

Brock was shocked, Stacy thought I was nuts, and Sean was thrilled. We named our new addition Rufus. How good it felt to have a new little (relatively speaking) life in the house. Puppies are great medicine.

As Sean's illness and the months progressed, I knew I had to choose between my businesses or my son. Of course, there was no choice: It was Sean.

Thank goodness for Becky Bone. Becky was from Perry, New York, just a few miles away from the village. When we decided to restore the old hook-and-ladder company in the village of Wyoming and create the Gaslight Christmas Shoppe, Becky was the first and only person I considered to help me. She was known in our county for her fabulous creative talent and could turn the most mundane things into works of beauty. I knew if I could talk her into going into business with me, I was halfway down the road to success. Luckily she, too, thought it was a great idea. I felt her creative talents and my marketing gifts would make us a good team. It did, and we put the Gaslight Village of Wyoming, New York, on the map. Characteristically, she came through to handle the business operations now, too. Between our secretary, Barbara, and Becky, the endless business pressures were under control.

One evening Stacy and Brock insisted that Brock and I go out for dinner alone. Sean was in a holding pattern, and they felt it would be good for me.

Stacy called from home an hour after we arrived at the restaurant. Sean had taken a turn for the worse. She tried to deal with him herself and called the doctor for help. Sean didn't want to spoil our evening either, but he was in terrible pain. I could tell Stacy was panicked.

We raced home from Rochester. I was angry at Brock and everyone for pressuring me to get out of the house. "Sean is is dying, and he needs me," I said. How could I have ever thought to leave him?

When we arrived home, Brock and I rushed so fast into the house that we both tried to get through the doorway at the same time and got stuck. Unstuck, we stripped our winter jackets off as we raced through the center hall into the family room where Sean's hospital bed was set up. Stacy heard us coming and rushed to meet us. As we all headed into the family room, she updated us on what was going on. She said Sean's pain levels had increased and he couldn't find a comfortable position. Nothing she could offer him was helping. She called the oncology doctor who was on call at the hospital, and it took him forever to get back to her. "Not only that," she said, "But when the doctor called back and I tried to explain to him what was happening with Sean he treated me as if I were an idiot. He was so condescending!"

As I was about to ask the doctor's name we reached the family room to find Sean sitting in the recliner chair we had brought down for him. He sometimes felt better if he could change position. "Mom, is that you?"

"Yes, Sean, it's Brock and me."

"I'm sorry I made you leave your dinner. I'm OK really, just can't get comfortable."

Trying to make light of it I said "Forget it. I didn't like the menu that much anyway." With that, he laughed, which broke the tension we were all feeling. It is remarkable how people who are suffering will do their best to make the ones around them feel better.

Sean was starting to get more comfortable and relaxed in the chair. Stacy reached out and touched his hand and kept looking into his eyes. "Thanks, Stacy," he said as she said her goodnights. Brock stayed with him for awhile to chat. When he knew Sean was feeling better he took his leave. I got Sean settled in his hospital bed and sat on the edge of the bed in silence for a few moments. I knew he would need his Ativan shot and I would stay with him until then. He was getting them every few hours around the clock now. The Ativan was a blessing. Normally used as an anti-anxiety medication, it is not meant to be used for long periods because it is very addictive. Now it is also used to help calm cancer patients. Coupled with morphine, Ativan helps control their pain and vomiting. Sean had been on large doses for a couple of months and needed it. He began to stir in his bed and his abdominal pain seemed to be increasing. He was getting ready to vomit. As I approached with his shot, Sean said, "Mom I hate to admit it but I feel so much safer when you are around. Maybe I get panicky when you aren't here. I'm sorry I spoiled your evening."

With tears in my eyes, I administered his shot and hugged him. "Flattery will get you everywhere with a woman my age."

EIGHT

STILL TRYING

Despite the puppy's cheery presence, Sean was in the wingback chair doubled up with pain. He couldn't hold much of anything down nor could he have a bowel movement. The doctors were telling him to take laxatives, but they weren't working. We were frightened, tiptoeing around, not knowing what to do, and hardly talking to each other, we were so tense over what would happen next.

Two days later I had shameful thoughts while shopping. I overheard two young mothers talking about their sweet toddlers, who rode in their side-by-side shopping carts. One was a sunny blond girl with eyes like saucers, about three years old. The other was a round little boy in overalls, about two. The women were chatting about preschool adventures and how the little boy almost fell down the stairs. Her friend expressed horror. "How could that happen; wasn't anyone paying attention?"

To my surprise I found myself feeling, *So what?* I had a sweet baby like you do and felt all you're feeling. We did all the things you're doing. Now he's dying. Twenty-seven years of mothering, of worrying, of joy and sorrow—for nothing. In fact, it is worse than nothing. Now I have all this pain and this suffering. I don't care about your children. Why should I care? It's too painful, too futile.

We'd been walking around with this giant weight on our shoulders. The sunlight seemed half-bright and our emotions and responses were muted. It was like living with gauze over our eyes.

Brock, Stacy, and I all felt it.

Two days later, Sean entered the hospital. Everything was happening so quickly and seeming to spin out of control. I even contemplated selling my businesses and devoting all my time to Sean. But, in the end, I realized there was no point to that. Life had to go on, no matter how painful.

All through this, Sean was wonderful. "I love you, Mom. I love you, Mom," he repeated every time I did something for him. Where was all his patience and courage coming from? His body was weak, yet his character was so strong. The whole family was inspired.

I sat with him a bit before he got tired. We no longer carried on what might be called conversation. I waited for him as he slept or watched TV or until something moved him to speak. He seemed to like having people he loved near him and sharing his space, just so he felt their presence.

It had been months since the experience with my foot without much discussion at all, when one day he asked, "Mom, do you really believe what happened to your foot was a message from God? I've been thinking about it a lot lately."

"Why have you been thinking about it so hard?" I asked.

"As best I can figure," he said, "God knows how much you love me. Maybe he wanted to comfort you while teaching me about faith? Maybe I must learn to put away my constant doubting and just accept things on faith?"

I looked at my son in wonderment. Could this be my avowed agnostic son talking? All I managed to say was, "Sean, I know it sounds trite, but God *does* work in mysterious ways. Do you realize that for the first time we are thinking about those mysteries together?" His silence was comforting. I was beginning to feel that Sean and I were exploring the possibilities; that as we were forced to take a path, a new blessing of understanding would be revealed to both of us.

I was forty-nine years old, and it still took me by surprise when people's lives took dramatic turns. The fact that my son had earlier decided to talk with a psychiatrist after years of never confiding in anyone had really floored me. And a bonus was that Sean really liked and trusted him. His illness made him realize how important it was to have someone to confide in.

Often it is the caregivers that cannot justify taking care of their own needs when ministering to the terminally ill. They tend to get caught up in the battle of life and death and forget that all good soldiers need to be healthy, rested, and well fed to win the war.

As the Easter weekend arrived I was increasingly angry with the hospital. So impersonal. So blasé. We were running out of time, and no one seemed to care.

Trying to distract myself and find some comfort, I watched every religious television special I could find. I watched with new eyes and listened with fresh ears. The real prospect of life after life had taken on new meaning for me, and I was convinced of the power of prayer. Again there was too much empirical evidence to deny the possibility.

Sean's pain was worse; he cried all day. I sent a message to his doctor.

Dear Doctor:

I am terribly scared! Sean is looking much thinner, afraid to eat for he binds up and has terrible pain voiding. His back pain is worse. I'm afraid if we don't do something soon it's all over for him. Please help!

Pam Yates

The doctor called with a report: CT scan—bad news. The cancer was advancing.

On April 14 we went to that hospital for the last time. The system had basically washed its hands of Sean. He met with several oncologists, each giving him the standard response: "We've tried everything we can, except surgery, and that would be very invasive with marginal results."

Sean was scared and distraught. Trying to keep our equilibrium, we asked about clinical trails. After all, this was a major cancer center. They said, "Sean, you don't qualify and, furthermore, you have to be ambulatory sixty percent of the time."

Furious, I found myself on my feet; yet I knew I had to control my response so as not to make it worse for Sean. I asked the doctor to meet me outside.

"It's April. He came to you last September, fully ambulatory. Why didn't you do something then? Why did you wait? I'll tell you why." I rattled on. "You had pronounced him dead before he even met with you and you've operated from that position since the beginning."

The doctor uncomfortably responded, "Mrs. Yates, there's no more we can do."

We had been spit out of there like a bitter pill. Sean was desolate.

I don't remember how we got to the car. I only remember Sean saying. "Mom, they didn't leave me any hope. What do I do now? This is supposed to be one of the best hospitals."

Brock and I fumbled for some words of comfort. How do you tell your son to give up, that he is going to die? We took him by the shoulders and looked into his eyes, "Son, this isn't the only place."

Sean responded, "I know there must be a doctor who will help me. I miss Dr. Bluming."

Brock drove us home. I could tell by his body language and facial expression that he was holding back the tears. I was terrified for Sean, who sat in stony silence. He gazed out the window. I could feel his emotional turmoil. I knew he was struggling to integrate what had just happened, trying not to think the unthinkable.

What could I do to comfort my child, this 6-foot tall man of twenty-seven years? I couldn't gather him up in my arms and cradle him as I had done so many times when he was young and hurt. What could I say? "Don't take it so seriously; this too shall pass"—that old standby expression used to assuage all the short-term problems of childhood?

Good God, we were there, we saw the doctors, we felt their hopelessness, we heard the formula responses, "We're done with him. Go home and wait."

I couldn't let Sean go home to no hope, to sit and wait for the end. I had to do something, but my emotions were overpowering my ability to reason logically.

I must have made ten calls the next day, networking like mad with anyone I could think of in the medical community. I got the name of a fellow member of the Chatterbox Club, a women's club that meets on Tuesdays for luncheon with various speakers. Her deceased husband had been a respected doctor in Rochester. Everyone said she was the one to talk to about a doctor who would treat Sean with hope and possibly different medicines. We all understood that at that point all the medications could do was to prolong the inevitable, but hope was the only medicine that could help him live out his remaining time with some peace of mind. And hope was something he desperately needed right then.

She gave me the name of a doctor in Rochester. She felt he had great humanity and would always keep trying new things for his patients until they could no longer tolerate it. His medical group was constantly working on new combinations of chemo, and he had spent many years at the National Cancer Institute before starting his own practice. She said to use her name when I asked for the appointment, and she wished us well.

Thankfully, there were so many wonderful people who cared and reached out to us during those terrible times. I knew to keep that in mind in the years to come and never forget how even the smallest gestures can be so comforting when you are hurting.

On April 20, 1994, Sean was admitted to the new hospital in Rochester. He was weakening as we entered that critical stage. There was no turning back.

I wondered if Sean would ever leave the hospital, but his hopes were high. The doctors had offered him what little hope was available to him. What he really knew about his fate was hard to tell. Once he was settled in his hospital room Sean seemed calmer. He was glad to be in a place he had confidence would help him. I knew he was nervous at home and felt vulnerable there. I must admit, Brock, Stacy, and I were relieved that he was there. We were scared and didn't know what else to do.

When we smuggled in the herbal mixture for Sean to soak his feet in, I wondered how the nurses would respond to our strange ritual. Of course a nurse entered the room just as Sean was soaking his feet. I've never been successful at sneaking anything. Amazingly the nurse remarked that years ago they always used foot soaks because absorption though the base of the feet is excellent. It seems it wasn't so crazy after all.

I spent the remainder of the day with Sean. Like him, I was getting to know the people and the system. While Sean went off for testing, I headed to the psychological and financial offices. I was glad he didn't know what we knew. Some doctors protested this decision, but I knew my son. He really didn't want to know. He needed the hope. I chattered nervously with him late that afternoon, trying to pretend this was just another day and we weren't where we were.

Brock arrived around five that evening and we all made small talk. Sean was very tired from his tests. Stacy arrived soon after. She looked uncomfortable seeing him. Sean's focus seemed to be on Stacy. He seemed to need to be close to her ever since he had taken ill. As children, their relationship had been strained. She was always good at everything, which magnified Sean's own lack of self-esteem. He also had channeled all his anger at his father toward her.

I sensed that Sean needed to talk with Stacy. I nudged Brock, and we said our goodbyes. Brock and I speculated about Sean's desire to be alone with her. When we met later she had obviously been crying. After an awkward moment, I broke the silence. "Did he want to talk to you?"

A little tear rolled down her cheek. It was obvious she struggled to keep her other emotions in check. She said, "Sean got up to go to the bathroom, and when he passed me, dragging the IV lines, he stopped, looked at me, and grabbed me, crying and hugging me. We stood there holding each other, sobbing while he told me for the first time ever, 'I love you, Stacy. I'm sorry I've treated you so badly. It was never you; it was me.' I didn't know what to say." Unable to find words to express our emotions, we sat together gently crying.

I tried to convince Brock to leave for Florida but he wouldn't go. It was the first year of the Cannonball Offshore Boat Race, a powerboat race from Miami to New York with major publicity and numerous entrants. He'd have none of it. I was so confused. Sean was excited and interested in Brock's going because this was one of the few things they could still share.

I told Brock that if he didn't go, Sean shouldn't know because it would scare him and make him feel worse to think it was because of him. For the next week we would have to play this stupid game of "Where's Brock now? Who's winning?"

April showers bring May flowers—was it really true, or like most other things I'd taken so much for granted all my life? The springtime had always been an almost euphoric time for me with its rebirth and renewal. As soon as the sun appeared, everything began to look better—fresher, cleaner. The heart gets a jumpstart and everyone is motivated. We'd always called it spring fever, the desire to dig in the dirt and get in touch with the best that nature has to offer.

On my daily drive I witnessed the passing of the gloomy and gray days of late winter, the mud and barren-looking landscape on sleepy farmland. The costume of winter that camouflages the rich, fertile land underneath would, in just a few short weeks, explode with new life. The fields all over the country were being prepared for the first season of crops.

This kaleidoscope of spring, with all its colors and new life, was set against a dramatic backdrop of the endless sky. I could actually sometimes be distracted from my pain and our personal drama in the presence of the mighty power that surrounded me on my daily sojourn.

Something greater than myself. That was an important concept to get my mind around. A miracle for all of us to enjoy. We take it so for granted. I promised I wouldn't ever again.

NINE

FAITH HEALERS AND FRIENDS

Sean's hospital room was empty and dark. "Oh no, he's dead!" I thought. Gathering my thoughts, I headed down the long hallway to the nurses' station. I had walked this hallway countless times to get to Sean's room. I didn't dare to look into the other rooms along the way, where patients lay in varying stages of illness. Fearing they would see my anguish, I never allowed myself to make eye contact. Once at the nurses station I was assured, "It's alright Pam, Sean has been taken to x-ray."

"X-ray. Why?" I was frantic. "Why wasn't I called?" I was furious at any attempt to patronize us or block our involvement in his care. It seemed that the medical establishment viewed me as a voyeur on this journey instead of as Sean's mother. Some seem to believe motherhood stops when someone turns eighteen.

Then I saw the bed being rolled toward me and I rushed to Sean. He had developed a fever and they thought the Hickman line in his chest had become infected. There would be yet another surgery to endure, if Sean agreed to it.

I looked from face to face trying to find some reassurance, but it was "business as usual" for the nurses and doctors. It wasn't until much later that I would understand that most doctors can't afford to get emotionally involved with their

patients. If they did, they couldn't face their day-to-day re-
sponsibilies. I looked at Sean in panic. Without emotion, Sean
consented to the surgery. I could see that resignation had set
in; he was just plain tired.

Late in the afternoon, Brock called from out of town. I
told him about Sean's condition. He dropped everything and
promised to be on the next plane. It was hard for Brock, too.
His life had to go on; we needed the money to help with
Sean's medical bills. My life now revolved around Sean. Everything else had to wait. And Stacy. She worked, went to
school, traveled to visit Sean, then headed home and started
all over the next day—always remaining stoic and not revealing much.

I walked with Sean to the operating room. He was so
vulnerable. How much can a human body take?

I kissed him gently and fought to withhold my emotions
and bridge the distance between love and detachment. The
anesthesia was taking effect—goodbye for now, my sweet
boy.

As I staggered toward the exit door, I turned to take a last
look and felt faint. Sean's surgeon rushed to catch me. He reminded me of Sean. I buried my head in his chest and sobbed
until my heart felt like it would explode.

The next day I arrived at the hospital early. I thanked
God that Sean was doing better but a small voice inside me
said, *perhaps it's too bad he survived.* How could I explain that
to anyone, wishing my own son dead? It is a conflict that only
those who have seen suffering can understand. I had seen too
many family members linger. Because I loved him so deeply,
I wanted it to end. The profound experience with the markings on my foot had convinced me that each soul goes on to
another life.

It was Mother's Day, but I didn't have time to think about
it. I had been too busy driving to Rochester to be with Sean
every day and, in addition, checking on my businesses. Brock
and I said goodbye that morning as we went our separate

ways. He was to spend the day with his mom at the nursing home as I made my usual pilgrimage to Sean.

Many days I didn't even remember the drive. My mind wandered during the hour-long journey.

That morning I peeked in on Sean and found he was sleeping soundly. I tiptoed back out just as a couple nurses approached. They wished me a happy Mother's Day. That felt like a low blow, but I knew they meant well. How strange to spend a usually joyous day at the hospital with your terminally ill son.

I sat on Sean's bed watching him sleep. Soon he woke up, looked at me, and asked how long I'd been there. Time had lost all meaning to him by then. I told him that I'd been there only a few minutes. He forced a smile and asked where Brock was. "He's gone to spend Mother's Day with his mother." As soon as I said it, I felt terrible. He started to cry, "Mom, I'm so sorry. I didn't remember. I didn't get you anything."

I hugged him, "Don't you know the best Mother's Day I could have is just to spend it with you?"

We held each other and cried.

Sean had been in the hospital three weeks by this time. It was hard to explain, but we had settled into a grim routine that sometimes almost felt comfortable.

Each day as I approached the parking garage, I would pray for a parking spot so I could get to see Sean as quickly as possible. Never knowing how I would find him, one nurse always gave me a hug while another updated me.

By this time I had begun to know the other patients on Sean's floor. Nearby, an old woman cried quietly alone. I'd never seen anyone visit her. Two doors down was a young man; his wife always tended him. I hoped the Lord had good things in mind for him because he had both multiple sclerosis and cancer.

I would find Sean, as usual, dozing in a drugged peace, and give him a hello kiss. The room was always dark; the light bothered him. His eyes would open and his day would begin.

Up to the bathroom, then into the chair for a smoke. He chain smoked, the only pleasure he had left. I could think of no reason to take his one physical pleasure away.

I shared news from the home front: Brock, politics, Stacy, the dogs, the businesses, news—whatever I could conjure up to make conversation.

And so it went. Doctors, nurses, aides, psychologists—our new world—but there was a measure of comfort in predictability. I sensed Sean felt that, too.

Sean slept most of the day. I sat and watched or paced the halls. The time went by. It was strange, with life ebbing away and time so precious, that we weren't talking about profound things. Just trivialities. It didn't make sense.

Heather Campbell arrived for a visit. It hadn't been so long since her daughter Kim babysat for Sean and Stacy. She was as close to a sister as I've known. Even though separated by distance, her love and commitment were a precious gift. I knew Sean would be glad to see her.

As Heather and I entered Sean's room, we found him sitting up in bed and smiling. He had just gotten off the phone with friends from Los Angeles. One called to say he was coming to Rochester to see him. Sean didn't have many friends, but the ones he had were extremely loyal. When Sean's cancer was diagnosed and he had to close his life down in Los Angeles and come back home, two friends drove his beloved black Mitsubishi Eclipse back east for him. It was his dream car. He had worked hard to buy it, and it always made him feel special.

Jacqueline Kennedy Onassis died on that day. We were all deeply saddened, Sean especially because he had been following her illness with great interest. Her struggle with cancer was personal to him. To Sean, as well as all of us, it was difficult to fathom the death of an icon. Only ordinary mortals like us can suffer such things. From Sean's perspective, if she could die from cancer, what were his chances?

The next day my mother arrived and we went directly to the hospital. I tried to prepare her for Sean's appearance. She hadn't seen him in a couple of months. A grandmother should never have to see her grandchild like that.

Sean would become the twentieth person on my mother's side of the family to die of cancer. Instead of hesitating she marched into his room without so much as a pause. She was an inspiration. I knew how horrible this was for her. She gave Sean a gentle hug and said, "Okay Sean. Nurse Nana is here. You'd better be a good patient." He smiled feebly. Obviously, he was glad to see her, but even a few minutes of interaction tired him out. He drifted off to sleep, and we headed for the waiting room.

As soon as we got to the small, sterile room with metal chairs, my mother began to cry. As I had anticipated, his appearance had shocked her. I was glad she didn't have to endure the day-to-day routine.

A friend had earlier recommended a faith healer named Uma. She was to arrive later in the day. Her coming visit fascinated my mom. Although Mom didn't believe in an afterlife, she was curious about all the alternative medicines and beliefs I was exploring.

We puzzled about what Uma would look like and exactly what she would do. I also brought the photos of my foot, desperately seeking opinions from anyone who might have seen anything like it before.

I decided to keep notes on each visit Uma made to see if there were any differences.

That afternoon heads turned as Uma walked toward the room. Mom and I were giggling and trying to figure out how Sean would react. Nervous giggling. We probably looked like we had lost our minds acting like that in such a serious place as the oncology lounge. It is remarkable how the mind's defense mechanisms kick in to help protect you from too much grief. Uma was a six-foot-tall, powerfully built woman. And she was wearing a turban. I resisted looking at my mother for fear we would burst out laughing. Uma was decked out in white from her turban to her shoes.

Uma extended her hand toward mine. She was blond with a fair complexion. Not the dark, swarthy, exotic mystic we had imagined. Her warm smile and quiet manner were calming.

We exchanged information and personal history. Uma had found her calling after years of personal growth through different religions.

A half-hour had gone by before I had the nerve to tell her the story of the markings on my foot and show her the photo. I continued to look for someone to solve the mystery. Uma was fascinated, "Why do you fight the mystery so much? Why can't you just accept what your heart tells you?"

I was startled. "I guess I'm afraid to accept what I know in my heart is true for fear I am pandering to what I want to hear."

Her face became somber and she took my hand. "Faith is simple if you're not afraid of it. The markings are what you believe they are."

She excused herself and headed for Sean's room. I stayed where I was.

Mom and I were filled with curiosity about how Sean would respond. We wouldn't have been surprised to see Uma come flying out vowing never to return. She emerged half an hour later, smiled and said he would have more energy now and be more comfortable. I pressed her for information. "Well, how did he act? Did he say anything?" She told us she asked Sean if she could come to see him again and he accepted. Wow! I was shocked that he had agreed. "Next week then," she said, and made her departure.

Mom and I hurried in to see Sean. He was sitting upright in the darkened hospital room. "Well how was it? What happened? Did you like her?"

"Yeah, I guess so. Nana, I felt kind of silly. I'm glad no one came in while she was here!"

"What did she do? Did she upset you?" My mother was concerned.

"No, Nana. She told me to lie still and relax and then she quietly walked around my body, from head to feet, waving her hands slowly over my body and spent a long time praying over my belly. It didn't hurt; it was relaxing. I didn't feel anything. Bad or good."

"You agreed to see her again, though?"

"It's okay Mom. I'll try anything. It can't hurt. Maybe there's something to it."

"My, my, Sean. You constantly surprise me. You're really opening your mind to new concepts. Very impressive!"

After a few minutes, to our surprise he got out of bed to sit in the chair and smoked a cigarette. He hadn't done that in days.

Mom and I didn't say a word.

Sean's hospital stay was in so many ways a comfort to all of us—including him. We all felt a lot less vulnerable and could escape the continual realization that he was dying. That did not mean that he was ever out of our thoughts. Everything blurred together. Each night when I returned home I tried to stay occupied. But often I could do nothing but raid the refrigerator. I had no heart for my usually creative activities, my enthusiasm having evaporated with Sean's illness. I'd been having trouble reading anything. My mind wandered, hopping from one fractured thought to another.

I must have pulled out a dozen books, reading the jacket covers in the hope that one of them would capture my imagination. Lots of good topics, but just as I'd think, "Yup, this is the one!" it didn't feel right. The second book from the left, top shelf, the one with the tattered black leather cover, caught my eye. It was Brock's old family Bible. In high school English class all the Protestant kids knew their Bible stories but, being raised a Catholic, I had never studied the Bible.

How wonderful! Brock's family Bible had all the family names down through the generations; it was charming. I took the Bible to my private sanctuary.

The next day Sean's closest friends in town, Jake and Sherry, visited. Since their teens, they had shared many ups and downs. Sean loved to be with Sherry's family. Even when he went off to seek his fortune in Los Angeles, a treasured part of coming home was the company of his best friends. I knew it was terrifying for them to see Sean so ill.

Ever faithful, Jake and Sherry came regularly to visit him. This evening they stayed later than usual. I think it got harder and harder for them to leave knowing his life was coming to a close. As they left we hugged. The grief in their eyes moved me to tears. I entered Sean's room to find he had already fallen asleep. I slipped into the recliner chair next to Sean's bed, watching him sleep as I had done so often when he was a baby.

The night nurse arrived. She was a lovely, gentle lady with delicate, fine features and prematurely gray hair. I'd seen her many times but never had occasion to chat. She called me out into the hall to reveal that she and Sean had developed a friendship. Wonders never ceased. He wasn't an easy talker and was quite shy most of the time. He seemed to have shared some family moments and personal information with her. I was glad. Maybe he was starting to open up to others.

She told me about herself. Her husband had died four years before. She spoke so tenderly I knew it was a close, happy marriage. He was a robust, active man, deeply involved with his family. They had a daughter he adored. His cancer had begun to take its toll and the doctors prepared them for his impending death.

Their daughter had wedding plans just three months away. Three months went by, and his condition became grave. He was determined to make the wedding, and to the doctors' amazement, he began to rally shortly before the special day.

She took my hand and sweetly said he stayed alive to see

their daughter married. He died a few days later. Choosing his time to die.

Suffering has a way of capturing time. As the months dragged on, there seemed to be a hundred hours in each day. I was watching my life roll forward in slow motion, much as a film editor, with a cut here and a paste there. Controlling the action to some small degree but never the essence of the story. A supporting player in an epic movie, that's what I was.

I couldn't imagine what the star of this movie, Sean, was feeling or how time moved for him. I was learning that, no matter how much you love or how much you try, you really have no control over the important things in life.

If you believe, as some do, that we are put here to learn our own personal lessons, then the fact that I could always make it better, no matter what the situation, was one of mine.

Images of Suffering

During the course of Sean's illness, I was told stories by nurses who believed, in essence, that each patient deals with mortality in his or her own special way. Many of them bore witness to patients almost dying and then being brought back to recall their near-death experiences clearly. Many nurses believe that when the end of life comes the soul has already begun its transition out of the body. Each person, they affirmed, chooses his own time to die and will hang on because he fears for his loved ones and has not been given permission to leave.

I witnessed that with Sean.

I learned that it is okay to let the person you love know it is all right to move on.

TEN

GOING HOME AGAIN

I arrived at the hospital a little earlier than usual. There in Sean's room was Ben Langley, his best friend since childhood. He was patiently watching Sean as he slept. I observed him for a short time as he silently kept his vigil. A good-looking young man, dark hair, clean shaven, just like my son should have been. One young man was in the prime of his life and another near the end of it. I felt tremendous sorrow as I watched Randy. The confusion and discomfort he was feeling for Sean showed in his facial expressions and the position of his body. He was shocked at the ravages that cancer had inflicted on Sean. It was probably his first encounter with death of this kind, the death of someone his age whom he loved. I admired his courage and caring desire to be there and show his love for his friend.

While Sean was still asleep, Ben got up without a word, touched his hand, and left the room. I pulled back from the door not wanting him to think I had been watching. He was a shy person and not very verbal. I pretended I was just arriving, and we exchanged hellos. He was overcome with emotion, but as our eyes met and I read what was in his heart, I knew he felt the gratitude that was in mine.

Driving home from the hospital in the late afternoon, I became obsessed with the desire to talk to someone of faith, someone who had experience with the life-and-death struggles of mortal men. There weren't many options. I had found no comfort at the abbey, and I could think of no one else to turn to. We didn't practice religion in the traditional sense, so I had no faith community to contact.

I felt a need to pour out my heart and thoughts. I'd always kept my own counsel or, in need, turned to Brock and sometimes Stacy. Not this time. This time I needed someone who could give me answers to my questions. I wanted truths, wisdom, and comfort.

Suddenly I remembered Father Robert Conlin from the small parish in Pavilion, New York. He was quite well known for his unique sermons and personality; and his use of theatrics was legendary. He would walk up and down the aisles of the church singling out men and women with personal references or stopping mid-sentence to tease a child. Father Conlin was fun, expansive, and eccentric in a charming way. Everyone was welcome in his church. He was a member of a rare breed of priests: trained in Rome, lovers of food, wine, and opera. Yes, Father Conlin would be helpful if he had the time.

I walked up to the rectory steps and knocked on the plain wooden door. Father Conlin answered and welcomed me warmly. He was aware of our family's travails and ushered me into the kitchen, where he began to sing a few choruses from an opera.

I made several attempts to tell Father Conlin what was on my heart, but he didn't give me a chance. He was seemingly uncomfortable with personal subjects. I realized that, even though a priest, he must have been one of those men who did not connect one-to-one, especially concerning unpleasant subjects.

I was disappointed, because I assumed a priest would be able to help me. I kept reaching out for wisdom and no one was there to help. Where could I find the answers and comfort I needed?

It was the second time I'd turned to men of faith for answers and comfort and been disappointed. Was it possible

I was never to find the answers I was seeking in people of faith?

I began to realize that what I was seeking had to come from within. As I trudged on through my sorrow, I was also becoming aware that spiritual and intellectual curiosity, coupled with an open mind, could possibly quench my thirst for the truth.

The mail had arrived by the time I returned home. With the usual bills was a wonderful gift from our friend Jim Atwell: a biography of Pope John Paul II by Tad Szulac. The inscription was very thoughtful: "Be not afraid." This from a man who had seen it all. He had been a colonel in the Army who served in World War II, Korea, and then completed two tours in Vietnam.

I would have loved to have gotten lost in a novel of pure fantasy, but I kept picking them up and putting them down. The titles turned me off. I just couldn't bring myself to read anything light. Our life was just too serious as it constantly revolved around life-and-death situations. So I decided instead to read the Pope's biography and was curious about his thoughts concerning the Virgin Mary.

After reading the book I got the idea to write the Pope and tell him my story and also include the pictures of my foot. I wrote a letter pouring out my thoughts and the story of the markings on my foot and held my breath as I put it in the mailbox.

Days turned into weeks and the grim trek from our house to the hospital became routine. Even though the life renewing quality of spring was everywhere, a rainy day affected my ability to cope with seeing Sean. Gloomy days dampened my spirit. I found it such work to get up enough courage to play the game of pretend for him.

It was a fairly routine day. He slept and I watched. The hospital was quiet. As usual, the nurses were kind and caring. They kept me posted on his progress. The night nurse told me Sean had asked about the nursery and expressed an interest in seeing it. I couldn't imagine what he was thinking, but I knew Sean; he would reveal his thoughts in his own time.

In May I had a meeting with Sean's doctors to find out the results of a CT scan. To everyone's surprise, it showed that the cancer had not spread any further. Brock was encouraged, but to my dismay I felt saddened. It only meant that the suffering would go on longer.

That day I found Sean sitting in his chair by the hospital bed, smoking the ever present cigarette and staring out the window. What was he thinking? I wished I could get inside his head for a while. His appearance gave me a start. I couldn't get used to this person he'd become—his gaunt face with days worth of stubble, the hollow eyes looking out of his emaciated face, his chalky coloring, and his arms and legs so frail. What had become of my handsome child?

"Well, Mom," he said. "How'd I do?"

"You did good, Sean. Frankly, we were all amazed."

"What do you mean, amazed?"

"We weren't sure the new chemo would work."

He got a little agitated with me. "Why didn't you tell me? I should have known."

As I looked up at him the tears filled my eyes. "We wanted you to be hopeful and not to worry. I'm sorry if we did the wrong thing."

It was a haunting encounter; a silent tear rolled down my cheek. Our eyes met, and with his long, thin fingers he brushed the lonely tear away. "Don't cry, Mom. It's no big deal."

What we were to learn next was a "big deal." Since Sean was now in remission he would soon be coming home. Unfortunately, the 24-hour care he required was not fully covered by insurance.

In early June, I met with the insurance coordinator and the patient release staff. I was there to learn how to care for Sean on my own. My head was spinning. To my surprise, his insurance would cover only four hours of registered nursing care a day and, according to New York State Law, only a registered nurse could administer the Ativan he needed. The Hickman line into his chest, the only civilized method of chemo and pain control, had a downside. We could administer the medications ourselves, but a licensed practical nurse in New York state could not. As a result I was about to become an instant medical health professional.

I met with the health care agency that would coordinate Sean's medicines and technical support and work with Wyoming County homecare nursing staff. The purpose of this meeting was for me to learn how to administer Sean's meds, give him his shots, and operate all the equipment. It seemed we were learning everything all at once.

That's what happens when the medical system reaches the end of its care options.

It's often said that, in the eyes of the insurance companies, you are only a number. In fact, Sean's insurance company had called while he was still hooked up to the chemo to tell the hospital that his allotted time was up and he had to be sent home. His doctors had to do battle with the insurance company to let him stay and finish out his treatment. Sean was released into our care, leaving us, like other unsuspecting families, with few options.

The only families who can afford around-the-clock care are the very rich. All others must handle the care with limited resources and options. I wondered how people who are emotionally or intellectually unable to cope can be expected to act as nurses. And what about the person living alone with no one to act as an advocate?

Before Sean returned home we converted the downstairs family room into a quasi-hospital room for him. The room that was once a warm, happy sanctuary, a gathering place for friends and family, had been transformed into a hospital room. Brock had Sean's hospital bed positioned in front of the TV for easy viewing, and the portable refrigerator was filled with

Ativan, saline, heprin, and TPN to keep him nourished. Sean hadn't had a bowel movement or anything solid to eat for two months now.

Sean was exhausted from the ride home. Wyoming County homecare nurses were there to coordinate his care plan and to set up a log we had to keep daily. We were to enter in all his shots, medicine times, dosages, and who administered them in this log. It is the law and is used to reference all information. Sean was agitated and barely uttered a word. I kept dancing around, trying to break the tension and fear we were all dealing with. The county nurses, while caring and helpful, were not well trained on the newest technology, such as CAD pumps and total parenteral nutrition or TPN, the liquid food that would be administered through Sean's IV lines into his chest to keep him nourished and alive.

Nervously Sean watched his new stream of nurses learn how to work the equipment. He was scared and it showed. I was paying attention, doing my best to bypass my own terrors at having to administer shots and TPN, trying to learn what to do without scaring him. A designated private care agency would always be available for help, but they were an hour away in Rochester. It was all like a bad dream. I couldn't imagine what Sean must be thinking.

Each day brought a new face, a new manner of doing things. Thankfully, we had the daily med sheets or I wouldn't have remembered all the names of the people coming to our home. For Sean it was like a revolving door. He never knew who would be tending to him. The nurses said he wasn't very conversational. Instead he was focusing on what they were doing and how well they were doing it.

Sean and I spent a lot of time just sitting together in silence. He had never been one to talk much anyway, but his pain levels and massive doses of meds made him groggy.

One of Sean's few areas of control was the television remote. The ability to make his own decisions was important to him. It helped him keep his dignity. It is important that terminally ill patients be aware of what activities they have control over. Anything from what flavor juice to the kind of mattress, the programs they watch and books they read, and also the nurses who attend to them, can be presented to them as a choice they can make.

I found again, like so many times in his recent past, that Sean was revealing parts of himself—ideology, ethics, and core beliefs—I never knew about. At one point Stacy came rushing into Sean's room, telling him to put the TV on. She was breathless. Before our eyes and the rest of the world, the O.J. Simpson Bronco slow-speed-chase on an L.A. freeway was unfolding. O.J. Simpson had been a hero of Sean's. He couldn't believe what he was witnessing. For the first time in a month or so he was involved and animated. His response, like most of the country's, was disbelief. As more and more information came out he started to doubt O.J. and then became angry. It was heartening to see him involved and passionate about anything at that point.

Options Even When There Are None

The most important thing I found with Sean is that control of his own life became tantamount. I made sure that he always felt that he had control over his life and decisions. Even when I feared for him and perhaps disagreed with his decisions, I forced myself to always keep in mind that his dignity took precedence over everything. You can bring terminally ill persons great comfort and peace by letting them take control of their lives.

Again, I stopped cooking. The smell of food being prepared would have been agony for Sean since he could no longer eat. We felt guilty sitting down to a meal while he was in the other room. Guilt, empathy, distress, grief—our emotions were all colliding now. Brock, Stacy, and I were having tremendous difficulty separating logic from emotion. Our hearts and minds were overflowing with the sense of impending loss.

Sean, on the other hand, was in a different place, responding totally out of character from what I would have predicted. He was processing his own depression, fear, and thoughts. It was as if he were watching and reviewing a movie of his own life. Grappling with the realities of his cancer and his suffering had brought him a new awareness. I knew I could only appreciate his state of mind when my turn came to cross over to the other side of life.

It was so selfish to say or think, but I must admit, and I'm sure Stacy and Brock would confess, too, that a part of me wished he were still in the hospital. I wasn't so frightened for him when he was there.

It was nearing the end of June, and Sean had been home almost a month. Brock, Stacy, the county nurses, and I formed the tiny circle of faces that made up Sean's world now. Everything around me—the house, the weather, Brock, Stacy, this beautiful summer day, the warmth of the sunlight, the garden filled with flowers of every color—it all seemed so normal, as it should. The phone rang as it always did. The dry cleaning was delivered every Tuesday. I shopped for groceries. It all seemed so normal, so predictable. Yet, lurking in the back of my mind and heart was the omnipresent knowledge that this would be the last summer he would see, the last year we would share, the last chance I would have to make his time better, to tell him I love him.

Worlds within worlds. How many at this moment, this glorious day, I often wondered, are also experiencing such sadness?

Why Me? Why Him?

I am proud to say that two of the most important
promises I made to myself at the beginning of Sean's
illness were that I would never wail, "Why me? Why
him?" I didn't because I know only too well that at
any given time all over the world there are millions
of people experiencing great suffering. I was never
alone and neither was Sean. I will be forever proud
of my son that, at least to us, he never said, "Why
me?" I believed I must honor his courage and do
the same.

Sean and I watched the movie *The Producers* with Zero Mo-
stel and Gene Wilder. Sean loved comedy and had a real understanding of what made it work. After reading books that
dealt with attitude during illness, he tried to watch things that
made him laugh. A movie was about the only thing left that
we could share.

When it was over, I hooked him up to his food and gave
him his shots. After a long silence he said, "Mom, you know
what? I don't think much about food or eating anymore. Funny isn't it? It was so important to me. I love the taste of things.
Now I don't care. It's like sex. I used to think of it all the time.
Now the memory of it stays with me, but the desire is gone."

It was moments like this that made my heart ache and
when the mother in me wanted to do everything possible to
ease his pain.

My late night talks with Stacy, on the other hand, helped
me more than they did her. I was getting to know her in a
way I probably never would have without Sean's illness.

In early July, Brock left on business for a couple of days.
The house seemed empty, and it was the only time I was
aware of the awesome responsibility I held in my care. I knew
he hated to leave, but life and work had to continue. I was
starting to realize the meaning of the old expression, "Life is
for the living." The world turns, the sun shines, thousands of

lives begin, and thousands of lives end—joy and suffering all existing in the same moments.

It was a beautiful summer day, as beautiful of a day that upstate New York could deliver. There was no humidity, just crystal golden sunshine. The valley shimmered in the sunshine, and the fields and grasses were verdant and lush. By all appearances, it was a glorious jewel to be relished. Thankfully, even in dreadful times, we have the capacity to appreciate the beauty and gifts of life.

When I checked on Sean he was experiencing a lot of pain. The cancer was progressing. *It* didn't take a holiday on beautiful summer days. It had its own sinister agenda. I bumped the morphine pump and gave him his Ativan shot and waited. No relief. I panicked but didn't let him see. After several minutes, when I couldn't control his pain, I saw fear in his eyes. I felt helpless. Hurriedly I went to the phone, my only link to anyone who could help, and called the doctor's office. The doctor advised me to bring Sean to the emergency room at the hospital in Rochester. That was the quickest way into the system.

It was a difficult task to get him dressed, into a wheelchair, down the front steps, and into the car. I grabbed the barf bucket, and all the medical cards, and drove an hour to the hospital. All the while Sean was in agony, and I was scared to death. Through it all I tried to act as if nothing was wrong.

We entered the emergency room, and it was filled with people of all shapes and sizes, with everything from the flu to a knife wound. The nurse asked me for the insurance cards. I told her Sean was already in the computer. She told us to take a seat, it would be awhile. She didn't seem to understand our situation. I leaned over the counter. My eyes were blazing. "Be awhile? He's dying of cancer! He doesn't have awhile. Take a look at him."

She looked at me with disdain. Then I said, "If you don't call his doctor right away, I'll take him through that door myself. So if you don't want an incident on your hands, do it now!"

She made the call, and soon Sean was placed on a stainless steel gurney and deposited in the hallway. What could they be thinking? He was loaded with cancer, his back pain was excruciating, and they left him there. When I asked, the nurse said there were no rooms available.

I began running around, talking to anyone who'd listen. Please, get him to a room, he's so sick. Everyone smiled but nothing happened. One hour. Two hours. Sean was suffering stoically. It was as if he was so used to agony he'd lost his will to fight.

But not I. Not ever. I couldn't imagine, or maybe I could, what happened to people who have no one to act as an advocate for them.

Who could help us? I thought about Father Norton, the hospital chaplain. A great, warm, compassionate man who, during Sean's recent stay in the hospital, always gave me good counsel. I took an elevator to the main floor where the chapel was located. I worried that he would not be in. I reached Father Norton's office just as he was closing his door on his way out. After I explained our dilemma he quickly followed me to the E.R. As soon as we reached Sean, Father Norton took one look at him and summoned a doctor. Within fifteen minutes Sean was on his way to the oncology department and a room. The nurses we'd known for so long instantly started to work on him, and between Sean's relief at being safe at last and the increased pain medicine, he soon drifted off to sleep.

God bless you, Father!

There was a new doctor in the department. He introduced himself to Sean and told us a bit about himself. He was a graduate of Vanderbilt University and new in Rochester. We were taken by his gentle manner and warmth. Sean and I wondered if it was because he was just starting out. Would he get colder after awhile, working in an area of medicine as difficult as oncology? Sean and I both agreed it must be so hard to do what they do and see what they see, but, thankfully, there are people to do such important work.

Sean seemed to respond to the doctor's youth and demeanor. I followed the doctor into the hallway to thank him. He hugged me and said the most remarkable thing. "Sean could be me. We are about the same age." I could see he was deeply touched.

Thankfully he was now in Sean's life.

After such a day I prayed that God would take Sean before he suffered more. I've known too many people who lost a loved one to pray for Sean's survival for my own selfish needs.

But I did have anger. My anger and rage were channeled exclusively toward the doctor back in Los Angeles. How could he have witnessed the disintegration of this young man and not been curious?

By mid-July Sean was back home and the daily routine had become a ritual. When I was busy elsewhere in the house, we used a walkie-talkie to communicate his need for pain meds. Every three to four hours he needed Ativan for anxiety and pain relief. As soon as he received the Ativan, he relaxed and dozed off. He had continual morphine in a battery-operated pump by his side. If the pain got too bad, he could "bolus" himself, a term for self-administered extra doses, but that was rare.

Sean had his own way of keeping score. He would resist increasing his levels of morphine until it got so bad he couldn't handle it. He felt that if his dosage was increased it meant he was getting worse. He wanted desperately to get better.

He also quizzed me. "Did you flush the lines? How much Ativan did you use?" I kidded him about not trusting his mother. We made it a game. Strange how your mind comes to terms with even painful things and your spirit finds a way to accept.

So much time to think; the days plodded ahead almost in slow motion. It was the first time in my life when I could predict where I'd be and what I'd be doing at any given time of the day. I was totally focused—no conflicts of interest, no tugs of guilt for things left undone, no desires other than to be there for my child. I found a strange kind of comfort in the total dedication and mission.

No Regrets

> We are all plagued with regret. My regrets centered around my lack of information. If I had known the questions to ask, I might have saved Sean from needless or extended suffering. Omission is a far different sin from commission, but you can be plagued by regret for things left undone. Be mindful from the very beginning that you will be left after your loved one passes on, left to replay the final days and moments you had with them. For your sake, as well as theirs, do all you can to make their transition as carefree as possible. In taking care of them, you will also be freeing yourself from guilt for the rest of your life.

On a sunny July weekend there was another attempt at normalcy. And another failure. We attended a small garden party social gathering in Rochester at a friend's home. It was a lovely evening, lovely people, all the elements that under normal circumstances would have spelled a satisfying experience—but I wasn't living a normal life.

Brock and I became separated. He was making small talk and I wound up in the kitchen with some of the women. The conversation centered around complaining about what an imposition carpooling was. It was all I could do not to blurt out, "Be glad you have a healthy child. Mine is home dying. Try having to take care of your dying child for a year. Watch him suffer and not be able to do anything to help. Now, tell me more about your problems."

I grabbed Brock, and we got out of there. There was no way I could be around normal people with normal problems right then. My job was to be with Sean.

It was a late July day, and I feared this would be Sean's final chemo treatment. He was so weak and his legs so thin and wracked with pain that the mere task of climbing the stairs to the tub upstairs to bathe and wash what little hair was left was too much. I even covered the mirrors so that he couldn't see himself.

We played games of "Later when I feel better." He always seemed to be so hopeful that I couldn't bear to be negative. It's all he had left, his need for hope.

I helped him into his wheelchair for the ride to the front door and his short walk to the car; then he endured the hour-long drive to the hospital where we put him back in his wheelchair for the ride to the oncology department. As I pushed him down the hall I saw how his frail, broken body melted into the vinyl of the wheelchair. He looked around as if in a daze. Was it the morphine, or was he looking at things as if trying to burn the images into his brain? I'd seen other terminally ill people with that strange stare, as if trying to hold onto the images of this world to take with them to the next.

We were greeted by all the nurses as if it was a happy homecoming. Their ability to turn grim into warm and cheerful was heartening.

Sean wasn't very responsive. He was exhausted, but he seemed glad to be there. I got him settled, and he asked for his bucket. He was vomiting every half-hour or so, more in the morning because the TPN liquid wasn't being absorbed into his body anymore. It kept him alive and supplied nourishment, but it also made his belly swell and caused pain. A terrible choice, but he couldn't stay alive without it.

He was more comfortable now, and I sat beside him. I stroked his forehead just like I did when he was a little boy. It still soothed him and made me happy. There wasn't much I could do anymore to comfort him. I felt helpless.

He opened his eyes and looked lovingly at me. My heart was aching and I told him, "Sean, you can never know how I love you and what seeing you suffer is doing to me." To my everlasting amazement (and he did amaze me often those days) he said, "Suffering. I'm not suffering like you think, Mom. I have to believe I'm going to beat it. You wouldn't give up, Mom. If you were where I am you'd have to believe."

We came home from the final chemo treatment. Sean cut it short. He was too tired and decided he'd try again later when he felt stronger.

I knew in my heart he would never have chemo again. What was I supposed to be doing or saying? I struggled to keep my equilibrium.

When Brock sat with him they talked guy talk—about superficial things, each trying not to upset the other. Stacy's visits were on a totally different emotional and psychological level. My role was to be his mother. I was also his primary, dispassionate healthcare provider and advocate. I hoped I wouldn't come crashing down from the pedestal on which he'd put me.

Stacy was on late-night duty. Sean seemed especially happy to see her. I tried to make myself scarce during those times.

One day near the end of July, Brock picked up his mother, Wreet, from the nursing home to come for a visit. I stayed home—Sean was too ill to be left alone. He needed shots so frequently.

Brock's daughter Claire arrived with her darling little Sarah, our first grandchild who had been born on June 6. Claire brought Sarah to meet her uncle Sean and her great-grandmother, Wreet.

Wreet beamed with pride as she held Sarah. Sean cuddled Sarah so tenderly even though it was painful for him. Claire took pictures that I know she'll always treasure. Brief, happy moments amidst unimaginable sadness.

ELEVEN

LETTING GO

On the first day of August we had dinner with some friends from Rochester, Scott and Liz Thomas, who brought another couple with them. To our great delight it was Rob Mazzilli and his wife Susan. Rob was about to become a senior executive at General Motors.

After the usual social exchange about children and their activities, the next hurdle to get over was deflecting the inevitable sympathies about Sean. I had learned to handle that conversation well. I had also worked very hard to learn how to lessen the terrible discomfort it caused those we came into contact with when they first learned about Sean's illness. Their pain and sympathies were written all over their faces. I had to try and remain calm and unemotional to get through these situations. Everyone had the best of intentions, but I knew I had to take the lead and others would take their cues from how I was coping. We exchanged niceties and then moved on to a subject more uplifting than Sean's disease.

While Rob, Scott, and Brock chatted, Susan—a serene, intelligent woman of great warmth—began to explain what she was working on. Along with her appreciation of the arts, she was working on a degree in the history of medicines and the evolution of cultural differences. The study of ancient tribes and cultures, their belief systems, and also their medicine interested her. I just couldn't get enough of her theories and ideas, which were fascinating.

After the men rejoined the group, Susan and I started to exchange theories about the paranormal. Her education about the topic far transcended mine. Reluctantly and with trepidation I told her the story of the markings on my foot. They were all interested and insisted I get the photos. As we looked at the pictures over dinner, all our friends confided that they believed in the paranormal; they all agreed that there was definitely more than our life here on earth. It wasn't a conversation you could have with just anyone. Susan asked if I had ever had a psychic reading. I said I hadn't, but since my strange experience I was very anxious to find a reader. She told a story of a personal struggle she was having. She went to see a psychic in Rochester and was extremely pleased with what the woman knew about her. I copied her name and promised I would give her a call. It was exciting, really, but that little voice again said, *Be wary, don't reveal anything—don't be a sucker.*

The more I opened myself up to different beliefs, the more I wanted to learn and read about faith. The little front bedroom had become my church. I had just finished Ian Wilson's book, *Jesus, the Evidence.* Words like love, peace, and faith were words we used so recklessly that they often lost their meaning.

The brand of faith that special believers like Peter and the apostles were infused with is a passionate, active force, a force so great that people are willing to die for a concept greater than themselves. That exceptional kind of faith must be lived everyday, not just spoken. I understood now that my trials and tribulations, my own personal tests of faith, were no tests at all compared with those of others. They were amateur tests with an amateur player—me. It was easy to claim faith in God and a great power while struggling with everyday annoyances. Faith is also a test of personal courage which requires letting go of yourself and your ego, and turning your life, as well as your intellect and your need for proof, over to a higher power.

It means that whatever happens, everything will be all right because it is part of a greater plan.

Some would say either you have faith or you don't. But I now believe faith must be worked on every day, just like marriage or anything worth having.

As the process of grief and the need to understand plagued me, I realized I had to let go of my son. I found I was conscious of a deeper faith evolving. Surprisingly, I felt closer to God and experienced more of a connection to and appreciation of all living things. I was firmly convinced that this life was no accident. It was all too exquisitely perfect and at the same time mysterious. I truly believed my own personal mystery was steering my life's course those days.

The early August nights were extremely hot and muggy. Sean didn't seem to respond to the temperature changes anymore. The bed sheets that he always wanted to protect him from being cold were now not used at all. Stacy and I shared night duty—11:00 p.m. to 4:00 a.m. My schedule at eleven was to hook Sean up to hyperalimentation or TPN, as those in the trade called it, administer shots, and spend a few minutes in conversation. I would give him the few letters he still received from those who hadn't lost interest in his struggle. But he didn't seem to care who called or wrote. Every night he just wanted to sit on the front porch in his favorite rocking chair, and have a smoke, and stare at the valley below. I could never have imagined how content this simple exercise would make him.

Stacy arrived home around 11:30 p.m. and immediately checked in with Sean. She administered his shots from 2:00 a.m. to 4:00 a.m. I didn't really know what they shared, but it was their private time. Her nursing and friendship had a special meaning for him, and I thought, for the first time in their lives, she truly knew he loved her.

Late nights were the only time Stacy and I saw each other. I thought she tried to stay away so she didn't have to deal with me and my feelings. While I tried not to be too emotional, it was hard. Over those last months, she had revealed more and more to me about her relationship with Sean throughout the years. I was surprised just how hard it was for her growing up, after I divorced their father, and how badly Sean had treated her. I'd learned much about her anger at Sean's treatment of her. He took out all his aggression about the divorce and his own feelings of worthlessness on Stacy.

Had I been too busy all those years ago with my new life to see what was going on right under my own roof? I thought I was paying attention. While Stacy found it confusing to care for Sean, considering their negative history, her compassion and love for him demanded she rise above it. She felt guilty about her anger toward him, especially when he was so vulnerable and was now trying to make amends.

Tension was growing. Stacy came home only long enough to relieve me and care for Sean. She was testy with me and expressed her need for privacy. When I would seek her out late at night to talk she seemed to get irritated. I wanted to talk with her, to feel close. She, on the other hand, wanted to be alone and not talk. Maybe my needing to talk and be close to her was driving her away. I was hurt, confused, lonely, but trying hard to understand. As it got more complicated, I found it was impossible to reach a level ground on which to operate. I didn't know what to do with the mother side of my life. It seemed too difficult for me and everyone else to deal with.

I talked to Brock and expressed my fears that I was losing Stacy. Frantically, I was trying to hold on to my family. While I couldn't save Sean, I had to save Stacy.

I decided to leave Brock and Stacy alone to talk. They always shared a bond and were alike in many ways. She didn't confide in others, deciding to keep her own counsel, especially now. It was easier for Stacy to talk to Brock, and I was grateful she had him.

Later Brock told me that his talk with Stacy left him unsettled. She felt I was looking for her to forgive Sean for the cruel way he had treated her when they were growing up and was afraid I would lose sight of the truth and create a comfortable fantasy about him.

How complicated this was all becoming, all the loose ends of relationships having to play out in fast forward.

Communicate and Share

Be sensitive.

Our family did a good job, but it took me some time to get it right. Each of us had our own saturation point.

Your time to unburden yourself may not be the right time to unload on anyone else. Learn to be observant and read the other person.

Each of us processes grief and fear in our own way and time. Learn when to put your own needs aside for the sake of the other person. Try to time your need for sharing and comfort for when the other person is ready to bear his or her own grief as well as yours.

Be patient and listen to their hearts.

Sean sat in the recliner doubled up with pain. I was scared, but I couldn't let it show.

I called Dr. Bluming in Los Angeles. Even though it had been August of last year since he'd seen Sean, I just knew he would be there for us. He had told us earlier that he was going to a conference in Arizona, "Please, if you need to talk with me, I will give you the number where I can be reached. Feel free to call me anytime." I was grateful for his kindness. He had been a solid rock through everything and an inspirational professional who showed so much compassion.

I called, left him a message, and he called right back.

"Dr. Bluming, I'm so scared. I don't know what's happening."

He said softly, "Yes, you do Pam."

It was like being punched in the stomach. I fell silent. He was right, and I knew it. After a moment of silence I gathered my panic and emotion. "I know, " I said, "I just had to hear it from you. "

Nestled in my little spot on the canopied bed in the front bedroom, I looked around at the books and snacks I had gathered to sustain my nightly vigil. What was it about this room? It was like a suit of armor, protecting me from the glancing blows of reality. A place where I could go to forget. It was like a womb where I could withdraw from my grief. I realized this little spot was perfect for the frightened child I was becoming. Here I was not the mother, but an innocent little girl.

Midnight on August 8 Stacy was edgy and upset. We all were. The 24-hour duty was taking its toll. We slept in fits and starts. All our waking time was taken up tending to Sean's needs. His body chemistry was changing dramatically, and our fears were at a fever pitch. When we spoke to each other we were snappish and half-hearted.

I was worried about Stacy. She was crying and frightened about what was happening to our family. We were all fractured and frightened and wondering what would be left of us when Sean died. How could I tell her that I didn't know? At times, she even appeared angry at Sean for doing this to our lives.

Tough times. And the worst, I feared, were still to come.

I checked on Sean, who had dozed off. Stacy was in the kitchen. I'd been struggling with how and when to broach the issue of our relationship. It was something I had to resolve. I was learning that tomorrows hold no guarantees.

"Stacy, we need to talk." She smiled, but her body language revealed her desire to be anywhere but there with me.

"Mom, I'm really tired. I've got a paper—" her voice trailed off.

"Please, honey, sit with me just for a minute." We took our usual seats around the kitchen table.

"Look Mom, I know where this is going, and I don't know how to respond to you."

"Tell me the truth."

"I feel you are looking for me to forgive Sean for all those horrible years, and I can't do that. And I feel guilty because I can't. He's going to die, but I can't forget." We both got teary, but she was trying to keep control of her emotions for fear she would not be able to hold back.

I said, "Just try to look at his need to make amends with you as a gift. Hopefully then you will be able to feel better about yourself. Maybe as time goes by it will help you to put him in a different perspective. I'm not a hypocrite; I don't want to make more of him in death."

Revealing a little more of herself and relaxing a bit, she confided that if I'd asked her four moths ago how she felt about him she would have been angry.

"Now Mom, I feel sad. I'm not afraid of him anymore. I'm really glad I am able to help take care of him. If I hadn't changed my feelings about him to a certain extent, I wouldn't be able to do this for him. I'm really angry at him for dying—just when he told me he loved me."

The nights grew longer and harder. The realities haunted me every waking moment—a few bad hours here and a few good hours there, an occasional light in the darkness.

Each evening when I was alone and everyone was in their safe places I played a game with myself. I forced myself to find a good moment, some positive lesson in the day's events.

Some days it was hard to do, but if I tried, really focused, I could grab hold of something that was said, or learned, or experienced that was good.

On a sultry August day the humidity hung low over our beautiful valley, and the heat created a hazy, out-of-focus picture. Sean was feeling somewhat better. The pain in his abdomen was taking a small vacation, allowing his spirits to rise. How little it took to make him feel hopeful. A moment of freedom from pain, an extra hour without his shot of Ativan, and he began to feel again that he was going to be all right. How cruel, this brief tease. But I tried hard to enjoy his optimism.

He was changing so much. I didn't think he could look worse. His hair was almost gone, only thin wisps here and there. His baseball cap had become part of his anatomy. Even the shape of his head had changed. His complexion was gray and chalky, reminding me of the faces of the Holocaust victims that had stared back at me from the television screen.

Confused and still questioning, I returned each night to my little front bedroom haven. I often prayed to the Virgin Mary about the perplexing mystery of my foot and the strange markings. I was curious that after so many years of my simple, sporadic praying to God, the only one who filled my mind these days was the Holy Mother. I felt connected to her. This half-Jewish, half-Italian, lapsed Catholic woman with no particular linkage to any religion had found comfort and deep faith in Mary. In the daylight, I might still question what had happened to me, but in the darkness I had my faith.

I was writing down my moments with Sean. He revealed much now in short sound bites. He didn't understand how poignant his comments were to me and why I soaked them up like food and water. They would have to nourish me for many years.

My parents arrived. I would have done anything to save them the shock of seeing their grandson so frail and ill. It had been over a month since Mom had been here, but Sean had changed so dramatically that I was afraid she and Dad wouldn't be able to contain their grief.

They needed desperately to see him, and I knew it was important for Sean to have their love now. If he were to die before they spent some time with him, it would haunt them for the rest of their lives.

As I feared, their shock at seeing him—especially my dad's—was staggering. To their everlasting credit they handled it with great dignity and grace. One more thing that I've learned during this process is to never underestimate the strength and wisdom of the older generation. Such wisdom that only comes through life experience is strong medicine.

Sean was very glad to see them, and Mom took her place in his healthcare routine as "Nurse Nana." She was deeply touched and thrilled that she could help. The time she had with him provided her many memories of their bond to sustain her in the coming years. My dad dealt with his time with Sean very differently. Unable to face the realities of Sean's impending death, his visits were of a lighter nature, the usual banter of Dad ragging on Sean, and Sean's classic response, "Oh Papa." It wasn't until my dad was alone that the impact of what he wanted to deny would hit him. Thank goodness their visit would only be a few days. Let them remember him that way. He would be worse in the end.

One evening I picked up Brock's family Bible again and read from the gospels. Each writer offered his own version of what he had witnessed and what those events meant to him.

All of a sudden a light went on in my mind, and the wisdom of the religious historians I had come to know through my readings began to crystallize into a couple of overriding concepts. First, most of the historical and religious information passed down since the beginning of time was done through oral tradition. Committing stories to memory and then retelling the tale was how most of the ancient cultures passed on their values and ideas. Rabbis taught through such traditions, and that information was sacred. Therefore, the argument that the gospels were written so long after Christ had died and therefore irrelevant was in itself irrelevant. The men who wrote those stories were living in a time of oral tradition. Men and woman would have placed a high value on what they saw and knew it would have been passed down like all religious teachings of the time. An emphasis would be placed on making sure each and every detail was committed to memory accurately. A lie would have been blasphemy.

Secondly, by all accounts these were ordinary men who went through an extraordinary transformation. The foundation of their faith and new life's mission was built on the belief that truth, love, honesty, and decency toward all men and women was the way to heaven and the promise of eternal life. Why would all these men independently misinterpret what they witnessed in the person of Jesus? Why would they choose their death over life if they had not truly witnessed what they believed to be the truth? Why are the simple truths hard to recognize? Why do we accept the darker side more easily? It occurred to me that my faith was becoming more real to me.

I was walking the halls every night trying to stay awake, afraid I'd fall asleep. Sean needed us for his shots every two hours. I ate, read, and walked. Very few friends came to visit anymore. Sean had been sick for so long now that people almost took his illness for granted. The immediacy had long since passed. Dennis Bain or John Coleman still called occasionally, but Sean was too tired and weak to speak for long. People stopped calling, and I couldn't blame them.

I'd never been a good spectator. Emotionally, I was thrashing around hoping to find some way to gain control of Sean's illness, but I remained a passive witness to the events unfolding under our very eyes. It was torturous for a problem solver like me.

St. Paul, Jesus, the Koran—the list grew longer, and so did the stack of books beside my bed. I devoured them. Each night I said prayers that God would take Sean. Each morning came the hope that God had granted my wish. I sought answers and comfort everywhere.

Friends and Family

Profound illness will change the dynamics of personal relationships. People you have known for years may pull away and not respond according to your perception of what is appropriate. People often do not know the right thing to do and say.

If you feel a sense of rejection on the part of a friend, accept that many people cannot deal with illness or tragedy.

I learned that the friends who are there for you at times of great stress are the ones who most deserve *your* precious time.

It seemed I was praying or, should I say, having more conversations with God, those days. When you're young there's little time or need to talk with him. You and the world will last forever, or at least more years than you need to worry about.

All of a sudden, the years start racing by, putting complicated, painful realities in your path. Before you know it, the older you get, the more you become aware of how very little you know. You realize the need to develop a dialogue with a power greater than yourself. I was finding tremendous comfort in that. It really set my imagination afire, and I felt a lot of fear and confusion drain away. I'd taken to reading everything I could on religion, faith, spiritualism—not Catholic, or any particular doctrine, just the writings and historical theories of smart men and women who spent their lives in search of truth and perspective. It comforted me. It was a good thing to do at night when it was quiet and I was alone with my fears and loneliness.

Another blessing. The gift of faith.

Faith is a Personal Journey

> I believe that everyone who faces his own mortality comes to accept that life is a miracle and, therefore, there has to be a greater power and more than this world we know.

We were up around the clock. Stacy took the 1:00 a.m.-to-4:30 a.m. shift, Brock 6:00 a.m. to 9:00 a.m., I took over again until the county nurses arrived. Sean was still very aware of his medications and shots. He still didn't trust the nurses, but they were very caring people.

He could give himself the shots, but the Ativan he was addicted to made him sleepy, and he often dozed with a cigarette in hand. He'd already burned a hole in one sheet, and the thought of fire scared us.

A few people scolded us for letting him smoke and not putting limits on his smoking time. No one could know how those cigarettes helped to keep him calm. The nicotine must work with the other medications. It was the only pleasurable thing left to him. He hadn't eaten in five-and-a-half months, or had a bowel movement in six.

Sean was keeping a mental measuring scale. He resisted increasing his morphine, because with each level increase he realized he was getting worse—it was his way of gauging his decline. The thing he dreaded most was having to use more.

However, as his pain increased we needed to adjust the morphine levels upward. I knew how this upset him and told him how painful it was for me to watch him suffer so.

Once again, he floored me. Denial is a powerful force. He said, "Mom, I think God is making me suffer now so I won't have to later when I get older."

His statement unnerved me, but it's the first reference to God he'd made. Obviously, all of those hours of silent contemplation and aloneness were bringing him to a different reality. I was grateful and, in a small way, comforted.

His Ativan was needed more regularly now. He was losing more weight, if that was possible. He used to be cold all the time, but now his frail body dressed in his hospital gown seemed to melt into the mattress—no covers, no chill. I thought his internal body thermostat was starting to fail.

The television was on, and Sean was alternating between dozing and watching. I was sitting quietly, just to be near him. A documentary on World War II was showing—endless pictures of young servicemen between eighteen and twenty-four, fighting and dying. All of a sudden he said, "Mom, they're so young to die. I'll be twenty-seven. I guess I'm lucky I lived so long. Poor guys. So young."

I didn't know how to respond. It was one of many such moments to come.

"Yes, honey, they were very young."

Sean was worsening; he had terrible abdominal pain and increased vomiting due to the TPN fluid. His body couldn't absorb it anymore. He needed constant attention, and we were burning out. The strain was taking its toll on the whole family. Brock began to administering the Ativan, and it broke my heart to see him girding up to enter Sean's sickroom. Brock was so squeamish about anything medical, but he felt so left out, so helpless that it was better to have him help. It would serve him well after Sean's death. I couldn't let him live with any regrets. He'd never be able to forgive himself for not helping, and Sean would never want that.

As the end of August approached, Sean's condition was deteriorating rapidly. I was now on a 24-hour-a-day schedule caring for him. Even when Stacy or Brock would relieve me, I couldn't sleep. My days and nights were all confused. Even though I was exhausted, I didn't seem to have an off switch.

Brock, Stacy, and I were terrified that Sean would burn the house down with his smoking. We knew we couldn't take the one pleasure left to him away, but still we had to protect ourselves and the house. We had a family meeting and realized that even thought we dreaded it, it was time to call in hospice.

Dorothy Anderson was a friend who lived just down the road with her dear friend, Maggie Tackles. Dorothy was also one of the heads of Erie County Hospice outside Buffalo, New York. Dorothy knew of Sean's condition and would often call just to see how we were doing and if she could help in any way.

After our family meeting, I called her, weeping, "Dorothy, this is the hardest phone call I have ever made."

She answered, "I know, Pam, but I have been expecting it. I am surprised you didn't make it sooner."

Dorothy and Maggie were as different as day and night. Maggie was no-nonsense, tell-it-like-it-is, but extremely artistic. Dorothy was softer and quieter, a good businesswoman. When I was with her, I sensed in her eyes the depths of her humanity. What they did share was an outrageous sense of humor.

When Dorothy and Maggie moved to the village and I first met Dorothy, during the usual social ritual of "What do you do?" and "Where are you from?" we realized that we had both lived in the same place at the same time—White Plains, New York. I was raised there, and she worked there as a nun. Yes, a nun. She worked at St. Agnes Hospital, where my mother also worked as a volunteer. I'd never before met a nun who had given up her calling to reenter the real world.

She obviously didn't stray much from her faith and humanity. She headed the Buffalo Hospice and served her faith and concern for others in a different way. I was certainly glad she was with us.

I had put off this call as long as I could. We'd tried to do this ourselves because I knew Sean wanted only us around. I explained to Sean about the effects the TPN was having on his stomach. He listened in silence. I also asked if he would mind if we got hospice involved now—at least to give us some relief so we could sleep.

I always tried to ask his advice. All he had left in life were those few choices. We could at least accord him the dignity of being able to make them.

Dorothy said she'd been waiting to hear from us. She knew we couldn't go on much longer without outside help. Each family reaches its own breaking point. She had put hospice on alert and all the wheels were in motion. She'd have someone from Genesee Hospice Family Care in Batavia contact us.

Silence Speaks Louder than Words

Life has a finite frame. You will find the impulse to get into profound conversations about faith, spirituality, family.

Don't pressure your family or loved ones to talk about the larger issues unless they are ready and feel the need to talk.

Each person's need to deal with powerful issues will reveal itself when and if they are ready.

Sometimes just to sit and share the same space is enough to bring comfort to both of you.

August 29 was an anniversary of sorts. Exactly a year before Sean had made his first visit to the cancer center in Buffalo. Now, a year later, Sean would enter the hospice program—the final road taken by the terminally ill. Until just a few months prior to that, all my knowledge and exposure to hospice was a documentary I'd seen in my late teens, a black-and-white short subject film shown before the feature movie at the old Colony Theatre in White Plains, New York. I remembered vividly being extremely impressed by this revolutionary approach to death and dying, a wonderful social experiment started in England whereby a homelike situation could be recreated. The patients spent their remaining days drinking morphine cocktails, fulfilling their last wishes, and enjoying pain free days filled with positive experiences. I was thrilled at the concept. For a young girl it was a great way to integrate the death experience with the feeling that my young life was going on forever.

Hospice is the only solution covered by insurance, but you have to agree to die. In most states, the service is only available to those whose doctors verify that they have six months or less to live. And even with hospice care, the family remains the primary health care provider. Hospice provides home health aides for the patient, nurse aides, registered nurses, housekeeping services when needed, respite care for family members, and pastoral care (when requested) for both patient and caregivers. Because RNs are more expensive, they try to accomplish the tasks with as few as possible.

A young nurse, Sean's caseworker, arrived late that morning. I liked Cary Midla. She was softspoken, thin, well dressed and, as with almost all the healthcare professionals I had encountered during Sean's illness, tender and sensitive.

More forms, more bureaucracy. I understood the need for all of it, but it depersonalized everything, and it felt more like a commodities trade than the tending of a human life.

Cary explained that we were still considered to be the primary healthcare givers. If Sean were alone, hospice would not accept him. They were only able to give a few hours of care a day. How strange it seemed! The person who is all alone is truly the one who needs the care but is not eligible unless he or she agrees to go to a live-in facility. I expressed my shock to Cary and wondered how someone could possibly go through what Sean was going through without an advocate, someone who could run interference and pay attention to all the instructions, medications, and problems that are the constant companions of the terminally ill. She agreed but said there were no systems in place to serve that purpose, and that just recently a few hospitals and schools were recognizing this need and developing advocacy programs. How sad to think of all those people going through these experiences alone.

Cary advised that, generally, only people with a maximum of six months to live could be enrolled. They would provide only palliative care. The patient must agree to give up all lifesaving measures such as chemo, experimental therapies, and so forth. I interrupted, greatly concerned because Sean had agreed to discontinue the TPN with the hope he could resume it when he felt better. She looked a bit confused. I explained that Sean was not dealing with his impending death. He needed to feel that he was going to live. I begged hospice and the doctors to let him have his small measure of comfort and hope. We all knew it would be temporary, and that his body couldn't tolerate the TPN for much longer. Options, hope, small blessings—the only blessings.

Cary said she understood our feelings and thought it would be okay. We finished with the final paperwork and agreed to all the conditions. The final countdown began. As she was about to leave, she informed me that they were understaffed and they could not provide RNs until the thirty-first. I said it was okay.

Later in the afternoon, we discontinued the TPN. We all grappled with the implications of this decision. It was truly the beginning of the end. To take away your son's nourishment, the only thing keeping him alive, was an earth-shattering step. We had to make the decision while Sean was still totally competent. I say "we" made the decision, but Sean only understood that, without the fluid buildup in his abdomen, he would feel more comfortable. His denial mechanisms were so interesting. He never asked too much but just enough to feel he had some control.

He did ask if he could resume it when he felt better, "Mom, do I have to go to the hospital to do it?"

"No, honey, I'll start it again whenever you wish."

"Okay. Let's stop it then."

Brock, Stacy, and I were numbed by the reality of what we knew and united in the terror of Sean's impending death. We huddled in the kitchen, exchanging some fears. How will it be at the end? How will we feel about this house? Will we still be able to live here with all our horrible memories? Stacy startled us with a thought Brock and I avoided thinking. "Mom, I'm afraid of being an only child. What will this do to our family?"

We ended this momentous evening in silence, and the three of us probably felt the closest we'd ever been. My own thoughts drifted to all those billions of men and women who had faced death through the centuries. I'm every one of them at this moment, alone with myself, no one able to do this for me. So weak yet so strong! A calm settled over me. The final battle had begun. Were we ready? We had to be ready. Sean needed us, and this had become our only reality—the proverbial calm before the storm.

The mask of death, the smell of death, was overtaking him, but Sean's enthusiasm the next morning was contagious. He told me he was going to walk to the front porch and sit in his favorite rocker to look at the valley and feel the warmth of the sun.

From the loss of muscle and body fat, he experienced periods of being extremely cold. The sunshine washed over his body. He drew a deep breath and smiled the first smile I'd seen on his face in ages. Out of the blue he said, "Mom, I can't decide what I'd like to eat first when I get better."

I was stunned. I didn't know how to respond. I was intellectually and emotionally in one place and again he was in another.

Was it purely denial? Did he really not understand, or did he really believe he was going to live?

I couldn't explore the questions. How could I rob him of these moments? I gathered my thoughts. "Gee, Sean, in your position I wouldn't have a clue. What do you think you'd like?"

"I've been thinking about it a lot these days," he said with an ironic smile, which was so like his sense of humor. I also marveled at how differently he saw things than most—very bright, very deep. "Never thought I was much interested in traveling the world, but I'd like to visit different cultures and experience their cuisines."

"Well, what countries intrigue you?"

"I was amazed how much you enjoyed New Orleans and tried Cajun and Creole cooking. I must admit I was a bit bent out of shape when you raved about the food."

"Typical brat kid. Wouldn't try foods when I cooked them."

Sean laughed and touched my hand. "You know moms have no credibility."

I said, "I know, I know. Well, go on, tell me where you'd go first."

"Maybe to Lebanon or Morocco. I tried some of their foods in L.A. and they were great. Indian food sounds good too, lots of spices. Some great salads would be good. I've had sushi, not bad."

He enjoyed his adventure of pretending, and I was comfortable with his reality, though it must have been awfully painful for him.

Again, I was dealing from my perspective and he from his. The pretense was a pleasurable interlude to him, and that's all I cared about.

What saddened me was that he had discovered a life's adventure worth doing, and he would never have the opportunity.

Go Where They Are

During the last stages of life, your loved one will often express fears or opinions that you may disagree with.

Confusion and unsettled behavior are often a sign of the personal struggle they are grappling with.

Rather than try to debate or contradict them, go with them.

Reassure them that they are safe and that you understand how they are feeling.

Give them the peace they are looking for.

On that final day of August, I made plans with the caretaker at the Wyoming Cemetery. What did I know? And when did I know it? They say a mother's link with her children is almost mystical. I finally agreed.

Three years before, on a whim, I had purchased three plots at the cemetery. I'd always loved it there. The cemetery climbed up the lush hillside dotted with old, noble trees, their branches spreading out wide. Generations of families that lived at Farmstead had been buried there. I loved that link with our home. You could view the splendid Wyoming valley with its fertile fields and winding Oatka Creek. It was a gentle spot where the wonders of God's best achievements nourished the soul.

A plot for Brock, a plot for me, but why a third? I don't know—it just seemed that I had to do it.

As I pondered the "why" of it, my mind drifted back to an old argument I had with Brock many years before.

When he and I married, the only source of friction was my relationship with Sean. He was an emotionally needy child, a lost soul in many ways. Brock always accused me of overcompensating for him. I did and I knew it, but I could never exactly explain why. Finally one day during an argument I blurted out, "Because I have this terrible feeling he's going to come to a tragic end."

My answer had stunned not only Brock, but me.

What did I know?

TWELVE

SAYING GOODBYE

As the summer shadows lengthened, Sean's fragile life ebbed away. Now our journey together—with all its ups and downs, joys and sorrows—was coming to an end. Maybe we were learning to accept the gift of God's love without the trappings of superficial beauty and material wealth.

Maybe God was testing my faith in ways I could never have conceived. Would I pass the test? Perhaps. At least I was trying. He was affirming to me that the sharing of God's love is what life is all about. While I could not speak for Brock or Stacy, I felt they, too, had gained a greater understanding of themselves and the meaning of love.

Sean was feeling more comfortable. He wanted to start the TPN again. Each time he made another hopeful decision it shocked me. It reminded me anew how desperate he was to live and how terrified he was to die. All I could do was be there for him and let him feel that we were all in this together. Whatever he wished I would do, if it was possible.

"Mom, do we still have the TPN? Is it still good?" There was desperation in his voice.

"Yes, Sean, there's one left in the fridge and it's good." I thought to myself, *Thank goodness, it's still okay.* He would have panicked if I couldn't have hooked him up.

"Sean, you realize you may start to feel uncomfortable again?"

He became quiet.

"Mom, if I can't take the TPN," he paused, "I can't live on Gatorade alone, can I?"

I almost swooned at the implication of his question, but I kept telling myself that if I didn't get frightened he'd take his cue from me. I seemed to have become his barometer for emotions.

"No, honey you can't." He grew silent, and I finally found the courage to look up from getting his shots ready and face him.

"But I thought if I were really going to die I'd know. I thought you'd be bouncing off the wall and so emotional that I'd just know. Bummer." I went to sit on the bed beside him, struggling with what to say, and wondering if I hadn't served him well.

"Sean, I told you when you were in the hospital how much we all loved you and admired you for the courage you have displayed and your will to fight this. I guess you just learned something about me. We felt it was important for you to never lose hope or to give up." By now I was crying. "I hope I didn't let you down."

Again, with his great compassion and dignity, he reached up and stroked my cheek. "No, Mom, you did great. No one could have done better."

Now we were both crying.

The following morning the TPN made him sick, and we had to stop. Watching him realize the implications of that broke my heart all over again.

My most painful moments came when I knew he needed comfort from his fear. The limits of touch and verbal speech constrained me. I felt the need to climb inside his heart and reach him down deep where he lived with that fear and aloneness. But I was impotent and useless. The only medication I had left for Sean was a mother's love.

Later that afternoon I was desperate, trying anything to find ways to comfort him. How I wished I could take this cancer from him. I looked through several books. There had to be something wonderful I could say to him. I was finding nothing I felt he would relate to. Just as I was thinking I'd failed again, the photo of the markings on my foot fell out from between some pages. It was so simple, so obvious, so perfect. Thank you, God!

I entered the family room. Sean lay sleeping, a skeleton wearing a baseball cap. I wondered whether to wake him. I had to. There were too many things to be said.

I gently nudged him, and he opened his eyes.

"Oh, Nurse Mom."

"Hi, honey, look what I found." I pulled out the photos from my shirt pocket. He quietly looked at the pictures. "Your foot. I forgot about that. Mom. It's weird."

Looking directly into his eyes I said, "Sean, I swear I did not do this to myself. I have spent the past months struggling with it, trying to figure out the meaning, and I couldn't. When it first happened, you asked why it didn't happen to you. I said all I could figure was that you wouldn't accept it. I still feel that's true. At that time you were not ready, but I was.

"Now, after all the questioning and doubting, there is one simple conclusion. The markings were meant to comfort us in our fear and give us hope."

He looked at me, understanding the message, and then out of nowhere he said, "Mom, I think I'll try soaking my feet. I think I've got to try harder."

I took his hand and told him, "No matter what happens, if you live or die, you must remember we were given this special gift. We know to trust in the fact that this place is just temporary, and we do go on. There is more, and these photos have certainly sustained me over the past months. I love you, Sean." We hugged each other, and I placed the photos by his bedside.

As I started to leave the room, he quietly called to me, "Mom."

"Yes Sean?"

"I love you, Mom."

With each passing day the conversations were getting harder. His imminent death pressed on my mind, my heart, and my emotions. I could never be where he was emotionally, and I knew it. I'd never had any training for this. Each conversation was agony. Will I say the right thing? The pressure was getting to me. I was like a raw nerve, and I feared I wouldn't be able to hold together for him. At night I was afraid to go to bed, and in the morning I dreaded getting up. It was all I could do to be with him and keep my equilibrium during our visits. I'd lost my focus, and nothing seemed important. All that mattered was that I would be there for him. I was scared of how his death would play out. What if I wasn't up to it? What if I let him down?

The next afternoon Sean was chain-smoking cigarettes between the morphine and Ativan. Friends had smuggled in marijuana cigarettes. Because they were harder to come by, he would save them for when his fears and pain were too much for him to bear. Every once in a while, I would catch him lighting one or smell the specific acrid odor they omit. In each case, I would not mention it. He would never think to smoke one in my presence.

This was certainly not the time for moralizing. I was seeing what a dramatic difference that marijuana made when coupled with other medications. He relaxed and his vomiting slowed down. There was definitely something to it.

Once I decided to sit down next to him while he was toking away. He was startled and uncomfortable. I said, "Sean, calm down. I'm a big girl."

He smiled and relaxed.

"Honey," I said, "I've never really smoked marijuana. I tried it just once, long ago. What does it feel like?"

He took another, long drag, laid back against his hospital bed, and closing his eyes, said, "It makes you forget all your worries."

I responded, "What in particular are you worried about?"

Once again I was always looking to draw anything I could from his emotional storage box.

He whispered, "Mom, when you're terminally ill there's nothing left to worry about."

Later that night, Sean awoke from his drugged sleep and seemed agitated. He called me on the walkie-talkie and I came running.

"Mom, I'm in a lot of pain." I hurriedly administered the Ativan and a bolus of morphine.

Shots of Ativan were coming more frequently. I didn't know whether Sean needed them for physical or psychological pain. He seemed strangely calm and very introspective.

"Mom, how is starving to death not going to be painful?"

Without missing a beat I replied, "Sean, from all I've read and all I can gather from the doctors and nurses I've spoken with, the mind and body start to shut down to conserve energy. Blood and energy start to defend the vital organs. You'll get sleepy and relaxed and eventually sleepier and sleepier. They say the mind and body seem to prepare for death. It's like having an out-of-body-experience."

Was I really saying those things to my son so matter-of-factly?

My heart was pounding inside my chest. I tried so hard not to scream. *Stop, don't make me tell you these things!* Next question.

"What if I can't get to the bathroom myself?" The bathroom. His only source of dignity left, another personal way of keeping score.

"Oh, that's no problem. There are bottles to urinate in and some people are fine until the very end." More questions!

"What about the morphine pills I have left? There are quite a few, aren't there?"

Knowing full well what he was asking, I assured him that if I could be sure I'd do it right, I'd help him end his pain.

Reflecting on my answers, he said, "I only hope I get those few good days before the end. Some people do, you know."

I assured him he would, and we'd do anything and everything he liked.

"Maybe I will sit outside and enjoy the valley."

"Of course, that's easy. Honey, I'm with you. We are *all* with you every step of the way. We will never let you be alone, not for a moment. You know, Sean, I believe you and I have been together in other lifetimes. We're too linked to ever be apart."

I kissed his face. He said he was sleepy now and would rest. I knew he needed time to process his questions and my responses. I hoped I'd done right. I'd never really know though, would I?

That evening Sean had guests. His friends Sherry and Ben stopped by to see him. I knew how hard it was for them, but they made him so happy and he felt that the outside world hadn't totally forgotten him. I showed them in and then left the room.

I was grateful for any opportunity to have a moment of quiet with Brock to watch something on TV. There had not been much chance for that these past months. We all felt the stress and overwhelming sorrow in our once-happy home.

Around 9:00 p.m. I was watching a sitcom with Brock when thoughts of Sean began to needle me.

I rushed downstairs and into the sickroom just as Sean was getting into his hospital bed. He was alone and behaving oddly. His bed was in the up position, but his body was slumped forward. His baseball cap sat unusually low on his almost bald head. He was strangely quiet and having trouble breathing. I rounded the bed trying to get a take on what was happening, but I had not witnessed behavior like this before. I began to feel panic.

I wondered if this was the beginning of the end.

His eyes had rolled back in his slumped head, and the cap had slid farther down his gaunt face. I watched his labored breathing and grabbed his hand to comfort him. "Sean, are you all right?" What can I do for you?"

"Just be quiet and sit with me. Don't talk, Mom."

"Okay, sweetheart."

He continued pulling for air and struggling to breathe properly. I couldn't stand it any longer. "Honey are you having trouble breathing?"

"No, Mom, I'm having trouble living."

Around 11:00 the hospice nurse arrived for the nightly vigil. She came just as Sean's episode, whatever is was, passed. He was not doing well; he had a fever and was extremely anxious. His nurse checked his vital signs, and we were working hard to get his fever down. It would be a long night.

September 7 was my Mother's birthday. I was glad she wasn't here. It certainly wasn't a day to celebrate.

Sean's pain and symptoms changed dramatically. Stopping the TPN and coming to terms with his death had taken their toll not only on his body but his mind. He was completely withdrawing into himself. I felt his fear and sense of hopelessness. It hung all around him like a pungent fragrance on a humid day, heavy and stale. A sense of foreboding enveloped him. We found the sounds of our life changing—from brisk walking up and down the stairs and halls to softer, quieter, less jarring shuffles. We whispered our converstions.

Uma came for the last time. She spent her half-hour praying over Sean and predicted he would again feel more energetic and comfortable. Even at this eleventh hour, she was hoping for a miracle.

As Uma and I chatted in the kitchen, the hospice nurse came in and sat with us. To our horror she launched into a clinical lecture about the stages of death, using terms both graphic and gruesome. It was all I could do not to get sick right there in front of her. I don't why I just sat in silence and let her go on. It felt inappropriate and cruel. She didn't mean to be, but it was as if she were talking to one of her medical colleagues, not the mother of a dying child.

The nurse finally left. Uma expressed her anger at the way she had spoken in front of us. I thought maybe it was just I who was too shocked to say anything, but Uma was horrified, too.

That afternoon, when I told Brock how unsettling the conversation had been, he called the hospice agency and expressed his anger. He asked them never to talk like that in front of us again.

Amazingly, that afternoon after Uma left, Sean did have more energy. It was the first time he had the strength to sit on the front porch in days.

Miracles and the Paranormal

Do you believe?
I wasn't sure, but after the journey of our family
through these troubled times,
I came to believe.
I have no other options.

On September 8 at 2:00 a.m. I was spending the night with the hospice nurse, Kim, whom I had just met that night but already liked very much. She was an LPN sent by hospice because there were not enough RNs. I stayed up with her to administer the Ativan. We talked and then I tried to catch some sleep. But it was hard. I was too anxious. So I decided to stay up and go out early to run some errands. When I looked in the mirror, I realized how much I had let myself go. Maybe, I thought, I should pick up some makeup to cover the circles under my eyes. The funeral would be soon; I didn't want my son to think I looked like an old bag—at his funeral.

The next day—September 9 at 12:15 p.m.—Sean Keith Reynolds passed away surrounded by Brock and me, as well as his biological father and an LPN from hospice. Stacy had finally fallen asleep around 6:30 a.m. I was glad she was not present at the moment of Sean's death.

Sean's death and final hours were far from the death-with-dignity scenario so beautifully and sensitively portrayed by virtually all the medical agencies and professionals who had counseled us along our journey. It was that hope which had kept our fears from overwhelming us.

Unfortunately, our experience was quite to the contrary. The last twelve hours of our son's life were the very antithesis of that promise of death with dignity.

At approximately eight o'clock on the evening of September 8, after his biological father had arrived, Sean started to get highly agitated and become incoherent. What the nurses had been saying about the patient waiting for a loved one or hanging on for a reason seemed to be true. After exchanging a few words with his father, his body seemed to start to shut down.

We witnessed these changes and called the doctor because we were frightened and didn't know what to do next.

I explained Sean's symptoms and the doctor asked us to increase the Ativan two or three milliliters, if necessary. "If you can't get him here, I'll *snow him*," he said. *Snow him* was a phrase I had never heard before. Confused, I said, "I don't understand what you mean."

"Give him enough pain medicine to calm him and keep him from being so agitated."

I told him that we couldn't get an ambulance because it was an hour away and Sean was too violent. He said to notify hospice right away.

We called hospice and explained Sean's deteriorating condition and asked for help immediately. The nurse on call said she'd send the night nurse as soon as she could. Two hours later, two nurses arrived. The older nurse was the night supervisor, and she brought along a very young-looking nurse. It was a relief to have them there. We could finally take off our masks of dispassionate healthcare providers and devote ourselves as father, sister, and mother. These would be our last hours together, and we just wanted to show our love for him.

From the moment the nurses arrived things started to deteriorate. The older nurse did not administer enough Ativan to ease his pain. When we realized that fact we asked her to give more. She argued that the dose she had given was all that his chart allowed. We challenged and insisted she call the doctor. Grudgingly, she went to use the phone and when she returned she upped the morphine but administered no Ativan. We pleaded with her, but to no avail. By this time Sean was grabbing at thin air and throwing his arms about, trying to pull his IV lines out. Stacy begged the younger nurse to give him the Ativan. She said she couldn't legally do it; besides she had never seen anyone die and his violent condition frightened her.

Meanwhile, the older nurse would leave at intervals to make a phone call and return to bump the morphine. Stopping her once, I begged her to help, "This isn't right." She grabbed me by both shoulders and coldly told me to "Get a grip."

My ex-husband and Brock were wandering in and out of the room, checking on Sean, but they were so disoriented and emotionally exhausted they didn't know what to do but pace.

At 2:30 a.m., the older nurse announced that she was leaving and the younger nurse, who had never seen a person die, would remain. I was incredulous, and Stacy was angry and frightened.

We had waited all this time for this final moment and for hospice to make it less painful. Then I remembered that the hospice agency supervisor, who was a registered nurse, lived about five miles away. I found her number and called it, waking her up.

I was talking in rapid-fire fashion about the past hours
and Sean's condition. Before I could finish she said, "Look,
you haven't slept in days. Get some sleep and I'll be right
down."

"Thank you, he's dangerous and we're terrified. We need
help."

"I'll be there. Take something to help you sleep."

After the hospice supervisor arrived and stabilized Sean,
everyone tried to get some rest. I finally fell into a fitful
sleep.

Suddenly Brock shook me awake. "Pammy, Sean needs
you. The nurse says he may be getting ready to have another
seizure. She thinks he may be trying to form the words, 'Get
Mom.'"

"Another seizure? What do you mean? How long have I
been sleeping?"

Without giving him time to respond I raced to Sean's
side. As I entered the room, everything had changed. It felt
different. There was a stillness, a solemnity, that hung heavy
over everything. A chill went through me. I stopped in my
tracks and in an instant took a mental inventory of the room.
Sean was propped up in the hospital bed, being supported by
his father and a different nurse, the LPN who had come the
other night.

The nurse said she thought Sean was getting ready to
seize again. I remember being furious that they were talking
that way in front of Sean.

Then I saw it—Sean's worst fear—a catheter was in place.
I took a deep breath, gathered myself together, and shut off
my emotion button. When I looked into his face I noticed
his facial structure had changed dramatically. It was elongated,
sunken, with hollow cheeks and vacant eyes. All my life's experiences, all my love, whatever intellect and wisdom I pos-
sessed, would be necessary to meet the demands of these final
minutes. Could I be what he needed? *Please, God, grant me the
grace to do and say the right things for my precious child.*

"Sean, it's Mom, I'm here. I love you. I've always loved you."

Upon hearing my voice Sean's restlessness eased and he grew calm. *He heard me! He knew me! Oh, no, that means he must have heard what they were saying!*

All those months, all the pain, all the new thoughts, all the many people, and all the mysteries explored and unexplained had brought me to this moment.

I realized as I spoke those final words I was, at last, truly ready to let him go. I felt strange, and an eerie calm wrapped itself around me. Something was helping me to help him let go. As if in slow motion, each of us was responding to completely different dramas: his violent seizure, my calm and measured words. At this moment we were all, perhaps for the first time, really in the same place emotionally. I was ready to let him go, and he was hearing beyond the words what I was really saying.

"It's okay to leave, Sean. It's time to move on. I'm here. I will be all right. You can go now. There is no more pain, only peace. I love you!" With that he had a final seizure and was gone.

As I kissed his forehead for the last time and touched his hand, I became aware that he had been clutching something, I opened his frail hand and, to my amazement, a photograph fell to the floor—the photograph of the mysterious markings on my foot. Sean had been keeping it with him.

That simple prayer to the Virgin Mary in November not only had sustained Brock and me but, obviously, Sean as well.

Our gift, our own little miracle, the answer to a mother's desperate prayer.

The gift of more.

EPILOGUE

I went to Toronto with Brock and Stacy two weeks after Sean died. We were forcing ourselves to do something upbeat and normal, trying to find equilibrium. I didn't know how to get us back on track, so I purchased tickets to *Showboat* on a whim, thinking a classic, old-fashioned musical might be just what we needed right now.

The show was great, very upbeat. Stacy and Brock enjoyed it, and afterward we had a lovely dinner. The subject of Sean never came up, and that made me think we were all working hard not to speak of the bad times. I had been haunted all day with his memory—the first time since his death that I experienced such torment. I had this need to know if he was all right. I kept talking to him, beseeching him to let me know that he was okay. I had even taken my diary to the hotel with me. It was as if I didn't make an entry, somehow I would forget him. I had to come to understand that in my heart. It would take me a long time to really accept that I would never forget.

Two weeks later I experienced one of the mysterious moments that had not quite become the norm but were too frequent to discount. We went to our place in the Thousand Islands after our Toronto trip. I was still distracted by my need to know that Sean was okay. Brock suggested that I take a nap, that maybe I was distraught because I was so tired. I'd learned over the past year that good sleep did help to put things into better perspective. I took his advice and fell sound asleep. I slept for two hours and woke up feeling much better.

I entered the great room to find Brock staring at the river, lost in some reverie. My footsteps broke his thought and he turned and asked me to sit down. John Mullin had called to tell us something. I was puzzled because Brock seemed so serious. I hoped something terrible had not happened to anyone in John's family—I panicked easily these days, expecting the worst.

To my amazement, John Mullin had called to tell us about Dennis Bain and a dream Dennis had the night before. John told us that Dennis had arrived at work very upset. He needed to confide his dream to someone, and John was the one he chose to tell. Dennis is not one to have flights of fantasy, so John was anxious to hear what he had to say.

Dennis told John: "I was in a very deep sleep. A dominant image filled my sight; it was a white telephone on a desk. The phone rang and I answered it, 'Hello?' The response on the other end was simply 'Dennis?' but the voice was very familiar, and I instantly knew it was Sean. I responded 'Sean?' At that moment Sean's image appeared over the phone. It appeared as a soft circle cameo head and shoulders. Sean looked good. He was fit and trim, clean shaven, with neatly combed hair. He looked great! He looked like he did after he started working out and lifting weights. I asked him, 'How are you?' Sean enthusiastically replied, 'I'm great, I've never felt better!' He was beaming. Then I asked 'Where are you?' He answered, 'Heaven I guess.' Just then the image widened out and I could see that Sean was in a beautiful ocean setting. The water was deep blue. It was a perfect, sunny day." Dennis said he didn't recall any other people or activity.

He continued, "Sean was out on the ocean skimming across the top of the water as if he were water skiing without skis or a boat, just kind of flying on the water. As I watched him go, I suddenly felt the strangest sensation, a warm, tingling glow over my entire body. It was literally from head to

toe, and the sensation woke me up. I was still tingling as I lay
in bed."

Brock said that John, who had worked with Dennis for
years, had never seen him so moved. I sat there drinking in
what I was hearing, and for the first time that day I felt at
peace. The love and closeness Sean and I had always shared
had managed to bridge the darkness.

Two months had passed since John told us about Dennis's
dream. It made sense to me that it would be Dennis whom
Sean would choose to reveal himself to. He and Dennis were
kindred spirits. They each loved comedy, and Sean looked to
Dennis as a mentor. Dennis wrote for the Comedy Club in
L.A. Sean was hoping to learn more about writing comedy
and wanted to try his hand at it. Sean also loved Zoe, Dennis's
four-year old daughter. Zoe had a giant crush on Sean, too,
and had drawn him pictures when he was in the hospital in
California.

Dennis called, excusing himself for not calling sooner, but
the *Truckin' USA* crew had been on a location shot.

I asked him to repeat his dream about Sean.

"You know, Dennis, when you asked Sean where he was
and he said, 'Heaven I guess,' that would be so like him. Always the skeptic, he would never have just said, 'Heaven'; it
would have to have been, 'Heaven, I *guess.*'"

We laughed.

I told Dennis that we had been trying to get Sean to the
ocean where he wanted to be, but he had been too sick. Dennis got very quiet. I asked what was wrong.

"Pam, I never knew Sean liked the ocean. He only talked
with me about the mountains."

Now, I, too became silent. If *Dennis* had imagined Sean, he
would have put him in a *mountain* setting, where he thought
Sean wanted to be, not at the beach. Only *I* would have understood the ocean setting. Dennis and I both had chills. It
was indeed a message meant for me. We were both stunned.

He continued, "Aside from the obvious, there are two other interesting points about my dream. First, I never knew about Sean's true love of the oceans. He always talked to me about wishing to go to the mountains or the woods, but never the ocean. I had no idea that for the past year you were exploring ways to get him to the water.

"Finally, as you know, Sean loved comedy. There were certain films he could quote verbatim. Whenever a biography appeared on the Marx Brothers, or some other comedy greats, he made it a point to record the show. He also enjoyed coming to the tapings of *An Evening at the Improv*. In fact, he always wanted to read my *Improv* scripts and liked to make suggestions on what worked and what needed more help.

"Anyway, during the September *Improv* tapings, about a week after my dream, a comic was doing a routine about the decorating taste of religious southerners and said, 'They all have that wonderful picture on their living room walls of Jesus water skiing without skis or a boat.' I was floored. The idea of water skiing without a boat or skis is very unusual. I don't recall ever hearing or imagining that image before my dream. Then just a few days after, a comic was using it in his routine. Sure, it might be just a strange coincidence, but that's a *mighty strange* one in my book."

I asked Dennis if he would mind writing his experience down for me. I knew it would mean a lot to my family, especially my parents.

"And by the way, Dennis," I said. "If Sean calls again, ask him to call home."

This, Too, Shall Pass

As tired as I was of hearing the expression, now I know it's true.

Grief is a personal thing.

Allow yourself the time and space to deal with your
emotions.

Don't be upset with others around you if they do
not grieve the way you think they should.

They can't—they're not you.

My grief spilled out at unexpected times in snapshots and
sound bites. Unexpectedly, a moment would trigger a memory and a picture. Sometimes it took my breath away, but I
allowed myself a momentary tear and then changed the subject. It worked. Brock's mother, Wreet, passed on some great
wisdom to me. She realized when her husband died that after
two weeks her friends became uncomfortable with her public
expressions of loss. She said, "Allow yourself two weeks to
indulge your emotions and then pull up your socks and get
on with life, at least in public."

In my grieving, I experienced a strange phenomenon. I
never remembered Sean's birthday or the anniversary of his
death. At first I felt terribly guilty. How can a mother not
remember those days? Then I realize that those days have become unimportant. Somehow, the totality of his life has taken
precedence over that brief, awful time of his death.

Hope Comes in Many Sizes

It can be the thunderbolt in the form of a remission
or cure, or it can be a collection of subtle events that
raise your spirits.

I have seen so many people come through tragic
life experiences and leave faith in the dust because
things haven't turned out the way they wanted.

If we were all granted the things we prayed for, we would take everything in life for granted.

There would be no divine mystery.

It had been six months since I had written my letter to the Pope. I was like a starstruck kid when I got the mail and discovered a reply from the Pope (or, at least, his representative). It was thrilling to see that letterhead. I got goose bumps.

How nice of them to answer my letter when they must receive millions of them each year. The letter said that the Pope would remember Sean in a Mass. How wonderful! Sean remembered at Mass in the Vatican. Even for a truant Catholic that was a big deal. I was glad I was learning to follow my impulses. Nothing was too silly or too big to at least try!

I still called Dr. Bluming every so often, especially when the day was filled with sunshine and beauty. I called just to tell him that he was in my thoughts. Not many oncologists get calls to simply say "Hello, I'm thinking of you." He deserved that; he had earned it a million times over.

Although I remain a believer in the hospice philosophy and care, ours was not a good experience. Sean's last hours were needlessly horrific. Because of the lack of available registered nurses, one hospice nurse under-administered medications upon which he was dependent and caused him to have painful grand mal seizures. They were understaffed and, based on nurses' testimony during subsequent legal action, we believe they only took our case because of our prominence in the community and the potential memorial contribution that would result.

Two years after Sean's death and at the encouragement of several nurses from the Hospice Family Practice in Batavia, New York, we instituted two lawsuits against the hospice agency. We did not seek money but rather a correction in the system. We sued on behalf of Sean and also his family. Since all hospice patients die, no one is left to legally complain about the service. Yet hospice is the only heathcare agency that has a mission statement that promises care of both the patient and the family.

Even with the heroic efforts and great dedication of our attorney, Michael Law, and in spite of the nurse's statements, both Sean's case and that of our family's were dismissed from court.

The court dismissed Sean's case on a technicality when it ruled that our first attorney failed to serve some papers in a timely manner. The family's claims were dismissed when the court held that there is no law on the New York State books that gives the family the right to sue, even though the hospice mission statement made a commitment to the family members.

The real tragedy is that New York State, by dismissing the claims of the family members, does not recognize the rights of the only people who remain after the death of a loved one. Therefore, no one is left to enforce and ensure that a hospice gives adequate and proper care to a dying relative. The deceased's loved ones are left to remember the pain and feel the guilt for the rest of their lives with no recourse. The feelings of helplessness abide.

Laws governing hospice care vary from state to state. Family members should be sure to understand the capabilities and obligations of a hospice facility before they enlist its aid. The hospice cause is noble, but human failings are universal. If possible, seek references from others familiar with the services of local agencies. Often, more than one agency serves an area.

I am glad the inequities of life don't make sense to me because it confirms the fact that there is more than we know and more than we can know. I would have been the only person that would have known that at the end of his life Sean longed to be sitting in the warmth of the sun at the ocean's edge.

My personal growth as well as Sean's gives me hope that this tragedy had a higher purpose. Most of all, I draw comfort from the memory of that night so long ago when the desperate prayer of a mother was answered: "If only I knew there was more, I could let him go more easily." I never asked Mary for the life of my son. Only for the strength and belief that there was more than this world. If I could believe that, I could let him go. Those strange and wonderful markings carried us through to the other side, giving us hope that we would all meet again. I believe that those markings and the photos were meant for me to share with others to bring comfort and hope.

After so many years, I still pull out my diary from time to time to reconnect with those times. Even as horrible as they were, at least he was there to touch. I could still hear his sweet voice saying, "Thank you, Mom."

As the old saying goes, "Time heals all wounds," and, thankfully, my need to remember is ebbing. The mystery of the markings on my foot is always with me. I can't count the times I waited in bed during those horrible final days expecting (as the hypnotist had predicted) another unexplainable event. "If you did this to yourself," he said, "then as Sean worsens, you will act out again. These are never isolated incidents."

I have experienced no new mysteries.

ABOUT THE AUTHOR

Pamela Yates was born in Bronx, New York, raised by a Roman Catholic father and Jewish mother. The dichotomy between these two religions formed a spiritual foundation that helped Pam accept divergent ideas while constantly striving for more information.

As an adult, Pam began a career in advertising, while also singing and traveling with the Sammy Kaye Orchestra on the side. She eventually left her career, moved to Connecticut with her children, Sean and Stacy Reynolds, and married well known automotive journalist, sportscaster, and screenwriter of *Cannonball Run*, Brock Yates. They moved to Wyoming, a sleepy little village nestled in the verdant valleys of western New York. She and Brock began to revitalize Historic Wyoming, affectionately known as the Gaslight Village, helping it eventually to become one of the largest tourist attractions in western New York.

In 1993 Pam was faced with a situation that put her spiritual foundation to the test when her son, Sean, a 25-year-old television writer, was diagnosed with a rare form of cancer. Mother and son began the journey that all parents pray they may never take. Hers is also the story of finding the "peace that passes all understanding" on a road that, as it turns out, no one ever has to travel alone.